Contents

Part 1. The Basics   1

Questions 1–7 cover the background topics in ovarian cancer, including:

- Where are my ovaries? What do they do?
- What does it mean to have cancer?
- What is a cyst? Is it related to ovarian cancer? How do a complex ovarian cyst and a simple cyst differ?

Part 2. Risk Factors, Diagnosis, and Staging   13

Questions 8–19 discuss the risk factors and symptoms of ovarian cancer and detail how it is diagnosed and staged:

- What does it mean to have ovarian cancer?
- Are there risk factors for ovarian cancer?
- What are the symptoms of ovarian cancer?
- How is cancer diagnosed?

Part 3. Treatment of Ovarian Cancer   37

Questions 20–47 discuss your options for getting ovarian cancer treatment, including:

- How do I decide on where to get treated?
- Must the surgeon remove both ovaries if I am diagnosed with ovarian cancer?
- When can I consider myself cured?

Part 4. Coping with Treatment and Side Effects   71

Questions 48–64 discuss day-to-day challenges faced by ovarian cancer patients, such as:

- Will I feel terrible during treatment?
- What side effects can I expect from chemotherapy?
- Is depression common after treatment?

When I was diagnosed with ovarian cancer in 1993, the only information available to women like me was statistics about the poor prognosis. Most of us were gripped by the fear of what happened to Gilda Radner. There was virtually no useful information that helped women understand and learn about the various types of ovarian cancer, treatment options, or how to cope with side effects. Despite the fact that I was unaware that the changes in my body were symptoms of ovarian cancer, I was one of the lucky ones whose cancer was identified early. Women should not have to depend on luck for a cancer diagnosis. This disease truly was "silent." How I wish this excellent book had been available to me and the thousands of other women who were searching for answers to their questions, and most of all, for the realistic hope that the information in this book can inspire.

Receiving a diagnosis of cancer is extremely confusing and emotional. Thanks to the increasing attention that journalists, health and policy leaders, writers, and publishers are beginning to pay to ovarian cancer, more women are becoming aware of this once called "silent disease." With the recognition that ovarian cancer has begun to receive—and this book exemplifies the best of that attention—women will no longer have to struggle to secure information to make timely decisions. *100 Questions & Answers* will help lead many women into the age of enlightenment about ovarian cancer!

Don't get me wrong—this was not an era that we sought. However, once we find ourselves here, it is essential that we have the knowledge to navigate through the maze of medical terms, distinctions among therapies, and other health issues we never before confronted. This book does just that.

100 Questions & Answers discusses the new therapies, not available to women like me diagnosed ten years ago, that have helped prolong survival. It also helps the reader understand risks and risk reduction strategies so that healthy women can gain the knowledge which might help them lower their risk of ovarian cancer, or catch it in its earliest and most curable stage. With this and other information about symptoms and the importance of second opinions and surgery by a gynecologic oncologist, this book is essential reading for the general medical community—nurse practitioners, primary care physicians, and obstetricians and gynecologists, who often are the first people to see women with symptoms.

Finally, this important book provides useful references to other books, articles, web sites, and support groups and advocacy organizations, such as the Ovarian Cancer National Alliance. Together they offer women and their families educational materials, the latest information about treatment options, community resources, and opportunities to raise awareness about this disease.

In fact, just as resources like this book have dramatically changed how women approach their battles with ovarian cancer, so too, has the advent of a national advocacy movement that joins survivors, family members, and medical professionals in a united effort to conquer this disease. Like most movements, the ovarian cancer movement began at the community level, and was led by women who were determined to make ovarian cancer "silent no more." The movement got a big boost when several of these women gathered in Indianapolis in the spring of 1997 and determined that there was a need for "something more." And thus was born the Ovarian Cancer National Alliance—a national umbrella organization that unites the efforts of individuals and groups across the country to focus national attention on ovarian cancer. Because there is not (at the time of publication) a reliable screening tool for ovarian cancer, the Alliance has kept its main focus on public education. "Until there's a test, Awareness is best!" is our mantra!

Guided by a strong passion to raise awareness about the symptoms and risks of ovarian cancer, to fight for more research funds, to make sure women with ovarian cancer get to the proper specialists and receive optimal treatments, the ovarian cancer community has expanded in many communities across the country and given voice to this once "silent disease." Since the Alliance's founding six years ago, these national and local efforts have fueled a dramatic increase in research funds, expanded treatment options, and even an improvement in survival for women battling ovarian cancer.

Heartening, yes. But the Alliance and our supporters are far from satisfied. We urgently need a reliable, easily administered early detection tool. And we will continue to advocate for expanded research funds and more clinical trials so that the next edition of this fine book will include even more answers for women with ovarian cancer.

Patricia A. Goldman
President, Ovarian Cancer National Alliance
July 25, 2003

Cancer has no meaning in itself. Yet it can bring a message; open some doors, while shutting others. It can bring darkness to one's soul as it can teach to ask for the grace of light in one's life.

I was advised not to attach any meaning to the cancer. Yet I talked to it, asked it questions, felt it; was mystified by it, humbled by it, saddened and depressed by it; had my eyes opened by it; was awakened by it; felt terrified of it, ashamed of it, forgetful of it, angry at it, and grateful for some of the changes and people it brought to my life.

During the first months after my diagnosis, I became aware that it is different for everyone and that everyone must find his or her own path in coping with it, medically, emotionally, spiritually, and physically. In this way, I came to feel a kind of distillation process, of becoming more myself because I really had to learn to trust the paths that were open to me and with which I chose to work: my medical team, the medicines, and the meditation. Chemotherapy was part of the path I chose and, therefore, though sometimes I hated it, I tried to be grateful for it and to use meditation to guide it in doing its work.

I want to say that having cancer just sucks, and it does, but I guess as humans we struggle to find meaning in our experiences.

Coping with an ovarian cancer diagnosis impacted my marriage. We had been married for only a year and a half when I was diagnosed. I lost the ability to conceive and entered menopause in an instant. I took a long time to let myself grieve these losses. My husband has been a tremendous support to me, but it has been hard on us both, and I think that sometimes it is even harder on a spouse. I think for this reason that it has been especially helpful to have friends, especially friends who have shared the diagnosis, with whom to talk. Depending on my husband alone to provide a sounding board and support—I don't think anyone could support that weight. In groups, we talked about the danger of our caregiver's "burnout" and how important it was for us to have a place or friendships to talk about the effects of the disease and its treatments and to share insights and medical information.

I read early on about setting different kinds of goals to help one to get into the habit of planning. There were so many months when I was afraid to plan because I didn't know how I would be feeling. It has been a challenge for me to set short-term goals, and to accomplish them, and to start planning longer-term goals. Living with the illness and its aftermath has taught me to live in the present, but I have to admit that there has also been the element of fearing the future.

So, for me personally, this trusting and learning to plan, letting go of the fear and need to know—because really none of us ever know where we will be in the future—and jumping into making longer-term plans has been an exercise in faith and courage. It has also been a lesson in learning to live with contingency but to go ahead and live anyway. I'm learning to sail, have taken up skiing again, and am doing more traveling.

I went through periods where it was uncomfortable for me to leave the house because I felt safe there, as I felt safe at the hospital. However, I don't want to live my life in only those two places! At times, though, I found I needed the comfort that only my home provided. Now, a few months after chemotherapy, I am exploring ways to connect with others and the outside world because I feel now that in engaging with others, and in practicing giving, I will again find healing and hopefully will positively impact others.

Often times now, as my health is good, I become angry at little things or at chance encounters, and I wonder to myself: Did you learn anything? But being well can mean forgetting about what it is like to be ill, so maybe it's healthy to feel life's minor irritations. And as I write, in health, I am reminded how I am able either to block out or forget the worst parts. I wonder whether it is the mind's way of going on; if you remembered every painful episode in life so readily, it would be hard to move ahead.

A friend and I talked about living to 100 and looking back—how many years spent worrying? Would I be anywhere different now if I had worried more? It is good advice, even if initially hard to accept and hard to practice.

Having cancer nearly broke me. I am now, paradoxically, more fragile and stronger. For someone who did not always face difficulties in life head-on, there was no alternative here. Now I can view it through the lens of "chronic illness," through vulnerability, through awe in the power of people's kindness and the power of prayer. I've changed, I'm a little chipped and worse for the wear, and I am better.

What I'm trying to impart are some aspects of the journey that I have experienced. Who knows what another will experience? There will be difficult times but also times of wonder and love. There is the outpouring of love, prayer, and help that came from family, friends, work associates, medical workers, and strangers. There is the gift for me of learning again to pray, to humbly ask for healing and to learn to accept all this outpouring of love. It is a huge shock to learn these things via a life-threatening illness and, if I could, I would have preferred to be wakened in a gentler manner.

There are many stories to be told for any one person's diagnosis of cancer. I am always a bit surprised when I read over a report made by the doctor during a visit. This is my story, told from the medical point of view, as I think the doctors try and write objectively. But what I am experiencing is very different, and my story would tell about conflicting feelings of wanting to be cared for and wishing that I didn't need to be cared for; of looking to my caregiver as a partner, as one on whom I depend for strength and hope but one who I also know (this from a "behind-the-scenes" peek during an off-hour elevator ride) can be overwhelmed and could possibly even complain about patients or workload, just as I have complained about expediency of treatment or the side effects of drugs or have been just plain ornery when I felt that I should only be gracious and thankful for my medical care. There is also one's life story, which gets interrupted by illness, and the struggles inherent in reclaiming it despite, or in light of, the story of illness; and how it affects one physically, mentally, emotionally, and spiritually. My life took a radical, unexpected, and frightening turn when I was diagnosed with ovarian cancer. And I have come to see the wisdom in the idea that the question faced by the ill person is not only "What are we going to do about it?" but also "How does one rise to the occasion?"

Currently, my doctor and I use the paradigm of "chronic illness" to describe my state. This can be a helpful way to look at it but, when I feel good and healthy, I cannot help but have faith that I am cured of the disease. I don't know whether this outlook is a boon or a bane, but it is just the way I have to cope.

Right now, I am writing in health. Every CT scan and blood test brings its concurrent anxieties, and some days are very hard. But I am learning to ride the current and, as a friend analogized, not get stuck on either side of the riverbank. This is not to say that a troublesome test result or CT scan will not deeply affect me: It will. But I continue to have faith that I have more to do here on earth, and I pray that God agrees with me.

I have many to thank, especially my medical team at Memorial Sloan-Kettering: Dr. Richard Barakat, Dr. Don Dizon, and Dr. Stephen Soignet; nurses Julie Esch, Sandy Pezzulli, Christina Perkell, and Susan Freeman; staff members Helen Lee and Rupa Bhatt; and all the nurses in the gynecological oncology department who have provided me with compassionate and expert care. I also thank my primary care doctor, Dr. Red Schiller, and staff at the Institute for Urban Family Health who continue to provide overall care and support.

A special thanks to the staff at the art therapy department and patient recreation departments at Memorial and to the staff at the Creative Center for People with Cancer for encouraging, supporting, and enlightening my creative endeavors.

---

[1]Frank WW. *The Wounded Storyteller: Body, Illness, and Ehtics*. Chicago: The University of Chicago Press, 1995, p. 65.

I have been in and out (for one 2-year period) of treatment for 4 years, including three surgeries and three recurrences. During this period, my beloved older brother, Peter A. Gibbs, died of pancreatic cancer after an acute illness of 6 months. His memory continues to give me courage and strength in his lesson of faith, dignity, and grace. My work on this book is dedicated to him, and to my husband, William Lefferts Brown III, who has provided me with love and support throughout this, our journey.

My heartfelt thanks go to our families—parents Paul and Barbara Gibbs; Bill and Peggy Brown; sister Jane; brother Phillip, sister Susan, and their families; and the many friends and family members who have provided us with joy, strength, love, prayers, and more love.

Andrea Gibbs Brown
April 2003

When I was asked to write this book, I thought that it would be an easy task. As a medical oncologist specializing in the treatment of women with gynecological cancers, I have seen and continue to see numerous women in various phases of their illness, grappling and living with ovarian cancer. It has always struck me that these women—no matter where they are from geographically, whether they are wealthy, middle class, or poor—all have similar questions when it comes to the diagnosis of ovarian cancer.

I recruited my friend and gynecologic surgical colleague, Nadeem R. Abu-Rustum, to help bring a balanced perspective to this topic. Because surgery is an important part of treating this cancer, I felt that his contribution would be essential to make this book as complete, and therefore as useful, as possible as a resource for patients and others whose lives have been touched by someone with ovarian cancer.

Almost as important was to ensure that someone who has gone through this experience would be a contributor to this book. After all, the person living with cancer can be the person most able to answer the questions about it. I was fortunate to have Andrea Brown agree to do just that.

Ovarian cancer can be a very frightening diagnosis. However, I hope the take-home message to anyone who reads this book will be that ovarian cancer does not have to control your life. I believe that knowledge is power, and I hope that, through this book, any woman affected by this cancer will be able to approach this diagnosis with the knowledge to make informed choices, coupled with less fear, so that her efforts can be better concentrated toward fighting and living with ovarian cancer.

Additionally, I hope this book will serve as a resource to everyone affected by this disease, including the families, friends, and colleagues of all who have ovarian cancer. I think cancer is more than an illness one suffers alone: It is one that affects family and friends. Andrea discusses the isolation of an ovarian cancer diagnosis, the wanting to protect everyone from it, and even the shame of it. She tells how she has overcome these feelings and, by doing so, how it creates a new sense of communion, of intimacy. I think it is a lesson well learned.

Those of us who treat ovarian cancer like to think we are doing more than performing surgery or administering chemotherapy or radiation. Every day, women welcome me into their lives and, in the process, I get to know them and their families. It is much more than just treatment; it is a relationship that we all hope will extend through the years. The fact is: We can cure ovarian cancer, but even when we cannot, we can help you to live with it, too.

I am sure some parts of this book will be hard to read, as there are some questions that are difficult to ask, let alone answer, in a straightforward manner. What we have attempted to do is to anticipate the questions all women think about when it comes to ovarian cancer and, certainly, those questions my own patients confront as we continue to work together. However, although some of the topics presented here may be hard to read, we have tried to be as comprehensive as possible. Please do not assume that all of these questions will apply to you, nor will everything presented in this book be your foregone conclusion. I cannot emphasize enough that every woman with ovarian cancer is an individual, and that one's specific path during this disease is not the same as others who have walked before you, with you, or even after you.

And so this book is dedicated to all my patients who have inspired me and continue to be a catalyst toward the work I do in looking for a cure.

I also thank my colleagues at Memorial Sloan-Kettering—David Spriggs, Carol Aghajanian, Paul Sabbatini, Sibyl Anderson, Jakob Dupont, Susie Jun, Richard Barakat, William Hoskins, Dennis Chi, Carol Brown, Elizabeth Poynor, Mary Gemignani, Yukio Sonoda, Mario Letaio, Bhavana Pothuri, and Doug Levine. In addition, I would like to thank my nurses, Christine Perkell and

Susan Freeman, nurse practitioners Jane Duffy-Weisser, Dorothy Dulko, and Sandy Pezzulli, my assistants, Helen Lee, Joe Larkin, Carin Zelkowitz, and Jovanna Roman, and the staff of the Division of Developmental Chemotherapy of MSKCC and of Memorial's Tenth Floor for their input and guidance not only in this project but throughout my career.

I further dedicate this book to my parents, Millionita and Modesto Dizon; to my partner, Henry Stoll; to our daughter, Isabelle Dizon-Stoll; and to my four sisters, Michelle, Maerica, Precy, and Marie, for their love and support.

Finally, I thank my co-authors, Nadeem R. Abu-Rustum, MD, and Andrea Gibbs Brown, for agreeing to take on this project with me. It has been a fruitful collaboration, and I walk away from it with much more knowledge gained, and two more friends to keep.

Don S. Dizon, MD
April 2003

PART ONE

The Basics

What does it mean to have cancer?

What is a cyst?

What is a tumor?

More ...

1. Where are my ovaries? What do they do?

An understanding of basic female anatomy and the function of the ovaries is a good starting point for the following discussion of ovarian cancer.

The ovaries, fallopian tubes, and uterus are what make up a woman's internal female reproductive organs (Figure 1). These organs lie deep in the pelvis and are connected to one another. The cervix is the external extension of the uterus and, together with the vagina and vulva, forms the female external genital tract.

Each woman is born with two ovaries, located on either side of the pelvis and flanking the uterus. Other organs are located near your ovaries: the small bowel and the **omentum**; the bladder, which sits on top of the uterus; and the rectum, which lies under the uterus.

Omentum

fatty tissue that drapes the stomach and intestines.

The ovaries are where eggs are stored. The ovaries start to release eggs when girls reach adolescence, and their

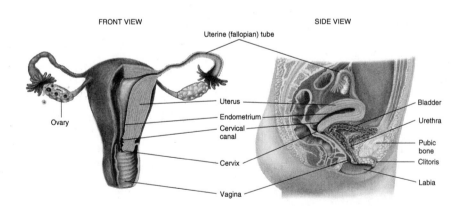

Figure 1 Anatomy of the female reproductive system. Reproduced from Alters S, *Biology: Understanding Life, Third Edition*. © 1999 Jones and Bartlett Publishers, Inc., Sudbury, MA.

bodies prepare themselves for possible pregnancy by the release of hormones called **estrogen** and **progesterone**. Eggs are released at monthly intervals (called **ovulation**), and their release begins the menstrual cycle.

The ovaries are essential as the home to those eggs until they're released into the fallopian tube and travel to the uterus. If an egg is not fertilized, the uterus sheds its lining. This process is manifest as **menstruation**, or your period. The ovaries not only carry a woman's eggs; they are also responsible for the release of estrogen that causes breast development and other sexual characteristics in women.

As a woman ages, the ovaries slowly stop producing hormones, which results in **menopause**. During menopause, the process of egg release slows down and eventually stops. In addition, estrogen production also slows. The uterus responds to changes in hormone levels and doesn't build up as much tissue as it used to, causing periods to become irregular until they, too, eventually stop. The symptoms of menopause occur owing to the gradual decline in the levels of estrogen produced by the ovaries.

2. What does it mean to have cancer?

As they do with other organs, a number of diseases and malfunctions can affect the ovaries. Cancer is just one of these. As we get into the discussion of ovarian cancer, we'll describe some common diseases that can be associated with, or sometimes confused with, ovarian cancer, such as ovarian cysts and **borderline** tumors (see Questions 3 and 4). First, however, it is most important that you understand what cancer is—and what it is not.

The Basics

Estrogen

a female hormone produced by the ovaries; it is responsible for female changes during maturity.

Progesterone

a female hormone made in the ovaries that normally works to prepare the uterus for pregnancy.

Ovulation

process of egg release from the ovary.

Menstruation

vaginal bleeding due to endometrial shedding following ovulation if the egg is not fertilized.

Menopause

gradual end to ovulation and menstruation that marks the end of a woman's child-bearing years.

Borderline

a term used to describe a tumor that does not appear normal but does not meet a pathologist's criteria for cancer; otherwise described as low malignant potential..

What Cancer Is

Cancer results when a cell starts to grow out of control. Normally, cells follow the same cycle of growth, cell division, and eventual death. When we were still developing, first as babies inside our mothers and continuing on while we were infants and children, our cells rapidly grew and divided. The end result was **differentiation**—it's what enabled a red blood cell to carry oxygen, an intestinal cell to absorb food, and an ovary cell to produce hormones to make eggs. If cells are injured or get too old, they undergo a process called **apoptosis**, or programmed cell death. This is what keeps us healthy and all our organs operating normally.

Some of our organs keep the ability to divide in order to replace dead and dying cells. These include the skin, gastrointestinal tract, hair follicles and, to a large degree, the ovaries, which replace their surface after an egg is released.

If a cell undergoes changes in its building blocks, called DNA, it can escape this tightly regulated life cycle. These DNA changes, also called **mutations**, can allow cells to keep growing and dividing. They no longer respond to your body's signals to stop dividing, and this process of unchecked cell division results in a mass of such cells, called a **tumor**. If a tumor cell breaks free from its origin (in this case, the ovarian cell within the ovary) it can travel through the bloodstream and land in another area of one's body far away (in the lung, for example) and start growing there; it is by definition **metastatic**. These two features—unchecked cell growth and the ability to metastasize—define cancer.

Differentiation

the process of cells maturing so they can perform specific processes in our bodies.

Apoptosis

programmed cell death.

Mutations

genetic changes in DNA; mutations are not always harmful but sometimes can be associated with cancer development.

Tumor

a mass of cells that grow abnormally.

Metastatic

adjective used to describe tumor that has spread.

What Cancer Isn't

It's important to state at this point that cancer is *not* something that can be passed from one person to another, like a virus or bacteria; cancer is not an infectious disease. You can't get cancer from another person, nor can you give it to someone else by simply coming into contact with that person, even close contact. A lot of factors contribute to the development of cancer, and having a family history of cancer is one of them. However, even if your mother had ovarian cancer, it doesn't mean that you will certainly also develop cancer— although you might have a higher risk of getting it than someone whose mother did not have it. Most important, cancer is *not* an automatic death sentence. That's a reaction many people have because, for decades, we lacked effective treatments for most kinds of cancers, and significant fear and stigma were attached to cancer. Thankfully, medicine has come a long way and, although cancer is still a fearsome thing, many people survive it, and some are completely cured. Innovations in treatment and new drugs are developed continually, so that even the most dangerous forms of cancer are becoming increasingly curable as new information about how cancer works is uncovered.

How Cancer Spreads

Cancer can spread in three ways: by extending into surrounding tissue; by passing through the blood supply, a process called **hematogenous dissemination**; or by traveling in the **lymphatic system**, the "cleaning system" of the body, in a process termed **lymphatic spread**. Knowing the ways in which cancers spread is important, as such knowledge is often used to decide

Cancer is not an automatic death sentence.

Hematogenous dissemination

a process of spread by which cancer travels through the bloodstream.

Lymphatic system

a network of lymphatic channels, lymph nodes, and organs, such as the spleen and the tonsils, that are the major component of the immune system.

Lymphatic spread

metastasis of cancer cells through the lymphatic system.

on what type of surgery is necessary and what other types of treatment are necessary (such as the use of chemotherapy and the number of cycles needed).

In the case of ovarian cancer, cells that line the ovary acquire genetic mutations that enable them to become cancer. Unlike many other cancers that tend to spread throughout the body, ovarian cancer prefers the environment within the abdominal cavity (also termed the **peritoneum**). Although it can spread to the liver and lungs or to other places, ovarian cancer is more commonly found growing within the pelvis or, when more advanced, in the abdomen. There, it can land anywhere around the abdominal cavity, surrounding the small bowel or colon, as a process called **peritoneal seeding** or **carcinomatosis**. These features are used in the staging (or classification) system for ovarian cancer (discussed in Question 15).

3. What is a cyst? Is it related to ovarian cancer? How do a complex ovarian cyst and a simple cyst differ?

A cyst is defined as a fluid-filled growth. Most cysts are not cancer and will go away if left on their own. Ovarian cysts are very common in women before menopause; however, they can also be seen after menopause. On the basis of how they look under ultrasound, computed tomography (CT), or magnetic resonance imaging (MRI), cysts appear in two types: simple ovarian cysts and complex ovarian cysts.

Peritoneum

the lining of the peritoneal cavity.

Peritoneal seeding

process of cancer spreading to involve the peritoneal surface.

Carcinomatosis

cancer deposits along the abdomen, often along the bowel and involving the omentum.

A cyst is defined as a fluid-filled growth.

Simple ovarian cysts are generally thin-walled and contain fluid. As seen on ultrasound, they have a characteristic appearance: They're bland, with a uniform wall around them; they do not have walls within them (also called **septations**); and they do not have differences in their internal appearance (also called **anechoic**). They're common and occur during egg formation, or **ovulation**.

When an egg forms, it forms in a follicle. If this follicle becomes big enough, it can be seen by ultrasound as a cyst (Figure 2); in this situation, they are often

Septations

thin membranes or walls dividing an area into multiple chambers. Often used to describe complex cysts seen on ultrasound.

Anechoic

used in ultrasound studies, it describes a lack of different ultrasound signals, commonly seen with simple cysts.

Ovulation

process of egg release from the ovary.

The Basics

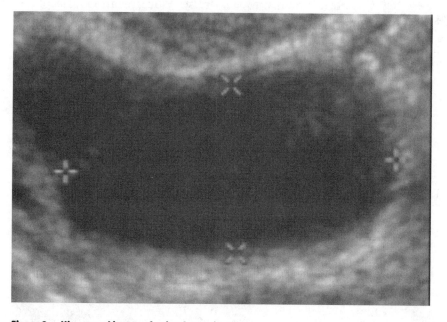

Figure 2   Ultrasound image of a simple ovarian cyst.

Theca-lutein cysts

functional cysts that occur in the ovary due to the cyclic changes of hormones during a woman's period.

Multicompartmental

multiple spaces, used to describe a finding seen in complex cysts seen on imaging studies, like ultrasounds.

Echogenic

an ultrasound term describing complex patterns seen within a cyst.

Papilla

budding formations on structures, seen on ultrasound or other imaging.

termed functional **cysts**. Cysts appearing this way are generally not cancerous.

Complex ovarian cysts are defined by the presence of internal walls within the cyst (septations) leading to the appearance of different rooms within the cyst (**multicompartmental**), different appearances within the cyst (**echogenic**), the appearance of buds into the cyst cavity (**papilla**), or differences in the thickness of the surrounding wall (Figure 3). Complex ovarian cyst walls may be thicker; they may show nodularity, a solid component, or debris. Complex cysts are more of a concern. They may be associated with cancer, particularly after menopause. Additionally, with special ultrasound imaging to assess blood flow (called Doppler imaging), these complex cysts may be found to be **vascular**, which may also raise concerns about the possibility of cancer.

The features of the cyst can best be determined by imaging studies, such as a pelvic ultrasound or a pelvic

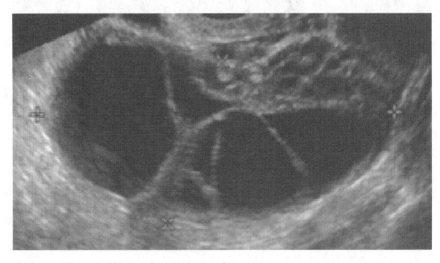

Figure 3   Ultrasound image of a complex ovarian cyst.

MRI. Depending on the features of the cyst as seen by imaging studies and on other clinical factors, a surgeon will make a decision with a patient whether to observe this cyst or to remove it surgically. Observation is commonly used in premenopausal women who have simple cysts or complex cysts that appear to be caused by hemorrhage or bleeding in the ovary, a common occurrence with ovulation.

Surgery is usually considered for large simple cysts that may cause symptoms of pain; for complex cysts with any of the previously discussed findings (papilla, multicompartmental, or thick-walled) at any age; or for complex cysts after menopause. Obtaining a blood tumor marker level, such as that obtained by CA-125 (see Question 13), may be helpful, but the test cannot specifically identify ovarian cancer.

4. What is a tumor? How do benign and malignant tumors differ?

A tumor is a mass of abnormal cells. To be specific, the term **tumor** is not synonymous with cancer. You can develop tumors that aren't cancerous, termed **benign**. The main difference between a benign tumor and a malignant tumor is that benign tumors do not spread.

In fact, most epithelial ovarian tumors are benign. Examples of these are **adenomas**. However, if a tumor can spread and invade, it is no longer benign and is considered to be **malignant**. A malignant tumor *is* synonymous with cancer. Pathologists refer to malignant tumors as **carcinomas**. The malignant counterpart to the previously mentioned adenomas is **adenocarcino-**

You can develop tumors that aren't cancerous, termed benign.

Benign

not cancerous.

Adenomas

noncancerous tumors arising from epithelial cells.

Adenocarcinomas

type of cancer, arising from the cells of epithelial origin.

mas, which are the most common type of ovarian cancer.

5. What is a borderline tumor? Is it ovarian cancer, or isn't it?

Some women go to their doctor with signs and symptoms of ovarian cancer, undergo surgery to remove the cancer, and then are told, "Don't worry about it; it wasn't cancer after all, it was a borderline tumor." This often results in more confusion and questions than even before the surgery.

Borderline tumors of the ovary do not appear normal through the microscope but do not have the appearance of cancer, either. They show evidence of increased growth and changes in their architecture that may not be considered normal to a pathologist. However, they differ from ovarian cancer because they do not show evidence of invasion into the surrounding ovarian tissue. Therefore, they're placed in an intermediate-risk group of tumors, which is why they're called **borderline** or are said to have **low malignant potential.** They are not, strictly speaking, ovarian cancer, but they're nevertheless an abnormality in the ovaries that can be harmful and must be treated.

Borderline tumors account for approximately 15% of all ovarian tumors. They require surgical staging just as ovarian cancers do. Although by their very definition they do not invade into the ovary, they do have the potential to deposit throughout the abdominal cavity, which is why they require surgical staging. In fact, their stage (see Question 15 and Table 4 on p. 25) appears to be an important predictor of survival and recurrence.

Stage I patients are likely to be cured at surgery, while those with more advanced disease are at greater risk of recurrence. Still, the prognosis of women with border-line tumors is quite good, with more than 85% of patients alive 5 years after diagnosis.

6. What is a dermoid cyst?

A dermoid cyst is the more common name of a mature teratoma, which is a specific type of germ-cell tumor (discussed in Question 8). Dermoid cysts are the most common type of tumor in young women and commonly present as an ovarian mass. They arise when a cell destined to become an egg starts to divide within your ovary, rather than dividing and growing in your uterus after it's fertilized. In the process of developing, such cells may also grow into different tissue types, such as teeth, hair, and even lung tissue. Cancer arising from a dermoid cyst is very rare, especially if it occurs in women below the age of 40, and surgery to remove the mass is all that's usually needed. Most women can expect to be cured after surgical removal of this tumor.

7. What is a Krukenberg tumor?

It might be confusing to be told that you have a cancerous growth in your ovaries, but you don't have ovarian cancer. The reason for this strange fact is that a type of cancer is always defined by *where it started*, not *where it's found*, which means that lung cancer found in the bones is still lung cancer, and breast cancer found in the liver is still breast cancer. This is important because different forms of cancer are treated with different methods: chemotherapy drugs that work against lung cancer, for instance, may not work as well against breast cancer or ovarian cancer, and vice versa. A **Krukenberg tumor** is cancer that's found in the ovary

Krukenberg tumor
a cancer that has gone into the ovary from another place, usually starting in the stomach.

but started in the gastrointestinal tract, and typically in the stomach. Because this tumor arose from somewhere other than the ovary, Krukenberg tumors technically are not ovarian cancer; this term is reserved for cancer that begins in the ovary. Treatment of a Krukenberg tumor is dictated by where it came from originally, so the treatments described in this book probably do not apply to patients with Krukenberg tumors. True ovarian cancer is described in the next section (Question 8).

Treatment of a Krukenberg tumor is dictated by where it came from originally.

PART TWO

Risk Factors, Diagnosis, and Staging of Ovarian Cancer

What are the symptoms of ovarian cancer?

What tests are used to diagnose ovarian cancer?

What is staging?

More ...

8. What does it mean to have ovarian cancer?

Along with the uterus and fallopian tubes, the ovaries comprise the internal female gynecological tract. As discussed in Question 1, the ovaries have two main functions: (1) the release of hormones that regulate menstruation and pregnancy and (2) the storage of eggs. Every time an egg is released, the ovary must repair itself and undergoes a process called **regeneration,** in which the surface is rebuilt.

The ovary is composed of three different cell types, or histology: surface or epithelial tissue; germ cells, which produce eggs; and stromal tissue, the mesh that supports the ovary. All three tissue types can give rise to ovarian cancer, but not all such cancers are treated the same way. This book focuses primarily on the treatment of the epithelial ovarian cancers, unless otherwise stated. Table 1 lists the types of *non*epithelial ovarian cancer.

Other types of ovarian cancer can occur beyond these, but they're much rarer. These types include **mixed**

Regeneration

to grow back.

Table 1   Major types of nonepithelial ovarian cancer

Histology	Percentage of All Ovarian Tumors
Metastatic	5–6%
Sex cord/stromal	5–8%
Germ-cell tumors	3%
Mixed mesodermal tumors	< 1%
Lymphoma	< 1%

mesodermal tumors (or **carcinosarcomas**) and **small-cell cancers**. The different types of cancer underscore the importance of tissue analysis by a pathologist.

Epithelial ovarian cancer is the most common type of ovarian cancer. It is a cancer that occurs in the surface (epithelium) of the ovaries and, as discussed in Question 9, is related to the frequency of ovulation. Although women of any age can develop it, most commonly it's diagnosed in women older than 60. Estimates claim that more than 25,000 women each year will be diagnosed with this cancer. Epithelial ovarian cancers can be classified further on the basis of the type of cells seen through a microscope. They are *serous* (most common), *mucinous, endometrioid, transitional-cell,* and *clear-cell* types of epithelial ovarian cancers. If a cancer bears no resemblance to any of these types of cancers, is it termed *undifferentiated.* The type of epithelial cancer generally does not alter the treatment plan, although clear-cell cancer may not respond as well as the others to chemotherapy.

Germ-cell tumors arise from the cells that produce eggs. Most germ-cell tumors are diagnosed in young women and make up 20–25% of all ovarian tumors, of which 3% are malignant. In 90% of cases, they involve only one ovary. Given that these tumors tend to appear in young women who may want to have children at some time, sparing the nonaffected ovary is a high priority.

Table 2 lists the different types of germ cell tumors. The most common type of germ cell tumor is the dysgerminoma, which represents 50% of all germ-cell tumors. The second most common is the **endodermal**

Mixed mesodermal tumors

tumors of dual origin with one part consisting of carcinomas and the other part consisting of sarcoma, hence their other designation as a carcinosarcoma.

Risk Factors, Diagnosis, and Staging

15

Table 2   Germ-cell tumors

Dysgerminoma
Endodermal sinus tumor (or yolk-sac tumor)
Embryonal carcinoma
Polyembryoma
Choriocarcinoma

Teratoma
    Mature
    Immature

Mixed germ-cell tumor

sinus, or **yolk-sac tumor.** The **immature teratoma** is the third most common, and prognosis with these is highly dependent on what they look like under the microscope; they are graded as low- or high-grade by a pathologist based on the amount of early nerve tissue seen in the tumor itself. Approximately 10% of germ-cell tumors will be made up of various types of tissue and are called **mixed germ-cell tumors.**

The type of germ-cell tumor that the pathologist finds under the microscope is a crucial factor in determining whether or not chemotherapy is used after surgery. Women who have had a thorough surgical evaluation and are found to have Stage I dysgerminoma or a low-grade immature teratoma do not require chemotherapy and have an excellent prognosis.

A lot of work has been done to identify what factors influence prognosis (prospect for recovery) in women with germ-cell tumors. A poor prognosis is associated with mixed-cell-type tumors; with large tumors (greater than 10 centimeters) that are made up of **endodermal sinus tumor**; with choriocarcinoma; or with immature teratoma. Tumors measuring less than 10 centimeters were found to offer a good prognosis, regardless of cell type.

Ovarian cancers that arise from the surrounding connective tissue of the ovary are called **sex cord-stromal tumors**. The cells that give rise to these tumors are responsible for the release of female hormones: estrogen (in the case of Sertoli cell, granulosa cell, and theca cell tumors) and progesterone (in the case of Sertoli-Leydig and steroid cell tumors). Sex cord-stromal tumors account for 5–8% of all ovarian tumors. The most common type is the granulosa-cell tumor. Because this type of tumor produces hormones, women tend to become symptomatic when the disease is present at an early stage. These tumors can affect both ovaries in 4 to 26% of cases, which makes a complete surgical evaluation very important.

The overall prognosis for women with sex cord–stromal tumors is very good, particularly because women tend to report to doctors early with these tumors. However, even in cases of early disease, the tumor can come back. It's not uncommon for women to have their cancer return after 5 to 20 years after their initial diagnosis, which is why close monitoring of women with such tumors is very important. These tumor cell types are included in Table 3.

9. Are there risk factors for ovarian cancer?

As with most other cancers, ovarian cancer likely arises from many factors and most likely is due to genetic damage that builds up over time. It is important to distinguish the difference between "genetic damage"

Endodermal sinus tumor

a type of germ cell tumor, derived from early cells destined to become eggs. Otherwise, they are referred to as yolk-sac tumors.

Ovarian cancer likely arises from many factors and most likely is due to genetic damage that builds up over time.

Table 3   Sex cord–stromal tumors

Granulosa-cell tumor
Thecoma-fibroma
Fibroma
Sertoli-Leydig cell
Leydig cell
Sarcomatoid (undifferentiated)
Gynandroblastoma
Unclassified

and "hereditary damage" in this context. Changes to one's genes, called **mutations**, occur spontaneously as a simple, random mistake in cell growth, sometimes related to an environmental factor. Most mutations are harmless; many that are harmful nevertheless do no damage because they are eliminated by the body's immune system, but some are able to escape the immune system, replicate themselves, and form cancers. A small number of these cancer-causing mutations can be passed from parent to child. Approximately 10% of ovarian cancer is truly related to heredity; the vast majority (90%) of ovarian cancers happen because of random mutations, otherwise known as **sporadic** mutations.

Several factors are associated with an increased risk for ovarian cancer. The most common type of ovarian cancer—epithelial ovarian cancer—appears to be related to how many times a woman ovulates. Every time an egg is released, the ovarian surface has to be repaired;

Sporadic

isolated; to occur without a pattern.

each time this happens, it creates a risk that genetic mutations will accumulate. This condition may lead to epithelial ovarian cancer. This hypothesis is supported by the fact that decreasing ovulation with the use of oral contraceptives is associated with a decreased risk of getting ovarian cancer in the future.

Other risk factors for ovarian cancer include older age, a family history of breast and ovarian cancer, and Jewish/Eastern European decent. The use of hormone replacement therapy (HRT) is not considered a risk factor. The use of fertility drugs for women having trouble with becoming pregnant has been debated as a possible risk for increased ovarian cancer, but no evidence concludes that these medications cause ovarian cancer.

10. Is hormone replacement therapy associated with ovarian cancer?

Hormone replacement therapy (HRT) has been used in women for several decades as a way to control the symptoms of menopause. The main reason for using HRT currently is to help to deal with hot flashes and night sweats associated with menopause. Although long-term use of HRT has been associated with a slight increased risk of breast cancer, HRT's association with ovarian cancer is less clear.

11. What are the symptoms of ovarian cancer?

One of the main problems with the diagnosis of ovarian cancer is that its symptoms are very vague. The main symptoms of ovarian cancer are bloating, abdominal discomfort, and distension, usually signs that the cancer has already spread beyond the ovary and even

Although long-term use of HRT has been associated with a slight increased risk of breast cancer, HRT's association with ovarian cancer is less clear.

into the abdomen. If bloating related to cancer is a presenting symptom, it is usually a sign of buildup of fluid (**ascites**) into your abdomen owing to the cancer.

Although there is no specific symptom for ovarian cancer, a woman should be cautioned that if she develops bloating, an increase in her waist line not due to a change in eating habits, lower abdominal discomfort, pelvic pain, discomfort during sex, or vaginal bleeding, she should seek consultation with a physician. Occasionally, women have shortness of breath that can be misinterpreted as a heart or lung problem; actually, it may be due to a buildup of fluid in the lung (a **pleural effusion**).

Acid reflux, constipation, nausea, or vomiting may also be obvious, particularly when associated with early sensations of fullness at meals or a generally decreased appetite.

It's especially important for women who are beyond the age of 50 and note any of these symptoms to contact their health care provider immediately and determine the cause of these symptoms. The symptoms may not be related to cancer, but if they are, the sooner it's treated, the better the chance for cure.

Women with germ-cell tumors often go to their doctor with abdominal pain that persists over several days or weeks and are also found to have a palpable (touchable) pelvic mass when examined. If the mass twists on itself or undergoes **torsion**, it can cause immediate and often unbearable pain. Such a mass can also cause pain due to bleeding or if it ruptures. These cancers typically grow very rapidly and at surgery can be as large as

Ascites

fluid build-up within the abdomen.

There is no specific symptom for ovarian cancer.

Pleural effusion

fluid build-up around the lungs.

Torsion

act of twisting or turning in on itself (ovarian torsion, for example).

40 centimeters. Fortunately, 70% of women with germ cell tumors will be diagnosed with early-stage disease.

Sex cord–stromal tumors appear early owing to their production of hormones, and their appearance can range from early puberty in young girls to post-menopausal bleeding in mature women. Abnormal vaginal bleeding is a common cause for women with granulosa-cell tumors to see their doctor. Other ways the disease can show up is by a mass felt on physical examination, ovarian torsion, rupture, or hemorrhage. Thecomas (tumors of theca cells) actively secrete hormones, and women seek a doctor owing to the effects of too much **estrogen**. Women with Sertoli-cell tumors also go to their doctor for the same reason, although they may have high blood pressure from excess production of a kidney hormone—called **renin**—necessary for blood pressure regulation. Fifty percent of women with Sertoli-Leydig-cell tumors notice symptoms related to too many androgens, or male hormones, and show up as a decrease in breast tissue or male-pattern baldness.

Renin

a hormone released by the kidney normally which is important in maintaining hydration.

Andrea's comment:

If you're reading this knowing already that you have the diagnosis, my thoughts here are not useful. But to those who are reading out of concerns for the future, I offer the following advice.

Make sure that your primary-care doctor gets all the reports from the specialists you see, and consult your primary-care doctor regularly. Report all your symptoms to your primary-care, along with your gynecological or fertility specialists, but make sure that one doctor you fully trust is seeing all the pieces of the puzzle. If you notice something changes in the way you feel, listen to your body, and make sure that you thoroughly impart these concerns and feelings to your doctors. If you're dismissed as healthy but still feel something is amiss, press on (there's something known as woman's intuition, after all). Sometimes, it can be easier to say, "Well, okay, if the doctor says I'm fine, I don't have to worry." I recall one gynecologist's office having a sign above the door: "Don't call us about lab results; if something is wrong we will contact you." Don't accept this. Always make sure you know the results of your tests and that your primary doctor has received and reviewed those results.

If your doctor does not take your concerns seriously, it may be wise to seek a second opinion (see Question 19).

12. What tests are used to diagnose ovarian cancer? How is a cancer diagnosis determined from these tests?

Ovarian cancer is diagnosed at surgery. Prior to surgery, tests that may help to make the diagnosis include a pelvic ultrasound (to check the size and nature of the ovaries) and a CT (**computed tomography**) scan of the abdomen and pelvis. Such a scan can show a pelvic mass and also describe the presence of ascites (fluid buildup) and the possibility of **peritoneal carcinomatosis** or liver involvement. An MRI (magnetic resonance imaging) of the pelvis is also helpful to describe the nature of any pelvic abnormality, especially how deeply involved a tumor is to its surroundings.

The main diagnostic tool for ovarian cancer, however, remains surgery. All the imaging tests

Computed tomography

otherwise known as a CT scan, this is a highly sensitive radiology exam used to help diagnose and follow patients with cancer.

Peritoneal carcinomatosis

involvement of the peritoneal surface with cancer, usually at the size of "rice granules" or tumor nodules.

22

described previously can suggest ovarian cancer.
However the tumor has to be removed, seen under a
microscope, and examined by a pathologist to confirm the diagnosis.

To make a diagnosis of cancer, a pathologist looks for
specific features in a cell. Some of the criteria that
influence a decision are (1) changes in the cell that
make it appear different from a normal appearance,
otherwise known as **atypia**; (2) intact or distorted
architecture of the cell; and (3) evidence that the cell is
dividing actively, also known as **mitosis**. A pathologist
can also look for evidence of spread, or **metastases**,
through the microscope by examining other tissue,
such as the lymph nodes.

A pathologist looking at an ovarian tumor may see the
cancer cells starting to pass through blood channels
(**capillaries**) or lymph channels within the tissue; that
may signal an increased risk for metastasis. In some
instances, the pathologist can make a diagnosis of cancer without needing to look at the tumor. If fluid was
surrounding the lung (pleural effusion) or was present
within the abdomen (ascites), analyzing the fluid for
cancer cells (known as **cytology**) could be sufficient to
make a diagnosis of cancer.

13. What is the CA-125 test and what is its purpose?

The CA-125 is a blood test that can be used in the
management of ovarian cancer. It measures a protein
(called an **antigen**) that is found in your blood stream.
It is a carbohydrate molecule (hence the CA, which
stands for **carbohydrate antigen**).

Atypia
used by pathologists,
it describes abnormal
cellular changes seen
under the micro-
scope.

Mitosis
process of cells
dividing.

Metastases
tumor that has
spread to distant
places in the body.

Capillaries
the smallest blood
vessels within your
body.

**Cytological
analysis**
the process of exam-
ining cells under the
microscope, which
are usually obtained
from floating cells in
the fluid of the
abdomen (ascites)
or chest (pleural
effusions).

Antigen
a protein that sits on
or is released from
cells that can be
targeted with an
antibody or vaccine.

**Carbohydrate
antigen**
a type of protein
released from cells.

This test has been available for many years but isn't considered a useful test to diagnose ovarian cancer. "Normal" CA-125 varies from woman to woman, so the measurement isn't an absolute, and fluctuations in the CA-125 level are common: it might be elevated one visit but below normal 4 weeks later. Such changes in the CA-125 suggest that other factors not related to ovarian cancer—endometriosis, pelvic inflammatory disease, and uterine fibroids, to name a few—can influence the CA-125 level. The CA-125 level is useful to help follow women who are being treated or followed after treatment for ovarian cancer and whose CA-125 was high at the time of diagnosis. That is, the levels of this antigen compared to previous measurements can be used as an indicator of what might be happening with the patient's ovarian cancer. If the CA-125 results remain low and within normal limits, it's usually a good sign that the disease is not back or growing. However, if the CA-125 value starts to rise beyond what the laboratory considers a normal value (in most labs, <35 mg/dL), a recurrence must be ruled out. Nevertheless, the CA-125 is not, and should not be, the only measurement for such tracking (or follow-up) in ovarian cancer. Remaining cancer may be present at a microscopic level even with normal CA-125 results, and it may take several months before a recurrence can be seen by CT (computed tomography) scan or MRI (magnetic resonance imaging).

The CA-125 may also be used in the initial evaluation of an ovarian cyst. A normal CA-125 result is often reassuring and may help your doctor to decide to observe—as opposed to operate on—an ovarian cyst. However, if the CA-125 result is elevated, it may be evidence that your doctor uses to recommend that an ovarian cyst be surgically evaluated.

Remember that the CA-125 (as mentioned) is not a test specific only for ovarian cancer, and its results can be elevated in a variety of noncancerous conditions, such as endometriosis, uterine fibroids, inflammatory diseases, other cancers such as breast or lung cancer, and even menstruation. This limits the use of CA-125 in ovarian cancer screening.

14. Should I have a PET scan?

A **PET (positron emission tomography) scan** is not routinely used in the initial medical handling of ovarian cancer. A PET scan remains an expensive imaging test that may be useful in specific situations, particularly in follow-up (tracking) of ovarian cancer. If a recurrence is suspected but can't be identified by conventional imaging tests, such as CT scan, MRI, or ultrasound, a PET scan may be helpful. It could be used to identify abnormal areas of uptake (absorption) that may indicate where tumor is located. However, at this point, a PET scan should not be routinely used for the initial identification of all suspected ovarian cancer. The role of the PET scan in the handling of ovarian cancer continues to be a topic of active research.

15. What is staging? How is ovarian cancer staged?

When you have surgery to remove an ovarian tumor, the surgeon will also check to see whether the cancer has spread throughout the abdomen and pelvis. This process is known as **surgical staging** (see Table 4).

Surgery for ovarian cancer requires a **laparotomy**, a vertical incision in the abdomen starting from the pubic area and extending to the belly button. The surgery requires removal of the **omentum**, the fatty tissue

Laparotomy

surgery through a large incision into the abdomen.

Table 4   FIGO staging system of ovarian cancer

Stage	Definition
I	Cancer is limited to one or both ovaries.
IA	Cancer is limited to one ovary, and the tumor is confined to the inside of the ovary, without evidence of cancer on the outer surface. No ascites is present, and the ovarian surface is intact.
IB	Cancer is limited to both ovaries without any tumor on their outer surfaces. No ascites is present, and the surface of the tumor is unruptured.
IC	Tumor meets the criteria for either stage 1A or stage 1B, but one or more of the following are present: (1) Tumor is present on the outer surface of one or both ovaries; (2) at least one of the ovarian surfaces has been seen to rupture (or ruptures during the process of removing it); or (3) ascites or abdominal washings are noted and contain malignant cells.
II	The tumor involves one or both ovaries with extension to other pelvic structures.
IIA	The cancer has extended to and/or involves the uterus or the fallopian tubes or both.
IIB	The cancer has extended to the bladder or rectum.
IIC	The tumor meets criteria for either stage IIA or stage IIB, and ascites or abdominal (peritoneal) washings contain malignant cells.
III	The tumor involves one or both ovaries, and one or both of the following are present: (1) The cancer has spread beyond the pelvis to the lining of the abdomen, or (2) the cancer has spread to the lymph nodes. The tumor is limited to the true pelvis but with histologically proven malignant extension to the small bowel or omentum.
IIIA	No cancer is grossly visible in the abdomen, and it has not spread to the lymph nodes. However, when biopsies are checked through a microscope, very small deposits of cancer are found in the abdominal (peritoneal) surfaces, also known as **microscopic metastases**.
IIIB	Deposits of cancer large enough for the surgeon to see but not exceeding 2 cm in diameter are present in the abdomen. The cancer has not spread to the lymph nodes.
IIIC	The cancer has spread to lymph nodes and/or the deposits of cancer exceed 2 cm in diameter and are found in the abdomen.
IV	Growth of the cancer involves one or both ovaries, and distant metastasis to the liver or lungs has occurred. Finding ovarian cancer cells in the excess fluid accumulated around the lungs (pleural fluid) is also evidence of stage IV disease.

FIGO = Federation International de Gynecologie et d'Obstetrique (International Federation of Gynecologic Oncologists).

that drapes between the stomach and colon; removal of lymph nodes from the pelvis and around the largest artery in the body, known as the aorta; and obtaining multiple tissue specimens (**biopsies**) from the right and left sides of the pelvis, from the right and left sides of the abdomen, and from both diaphragms. In addition, surgeons would obtain washings from the abdomen to assess for floating cancer cells. The appendix might also be removed. The pelvic part of the procedure requires removal of both tubes and ovaries and the uterus (**bilateral salpingo-oophorectomy** and **total hysterectomy**).

Biopsy

small amounts of tissue taken during surgery or a less invasive procedure for analysis by a pathologist.

Very few women get ovarian cancer before menopause, so retaining fertility is not a concern for nearly 90% of ovarian cancer patients—but there are occasionally younger women, like Andrea, who are diagnosed with cancer before menopause. In selected patients who strongly want to have children some day and in whom no visible disease is seen outside the ovaries at the time of surgery, a fertility sparing operation could be performed (see Question 24).

Bilateral salpingo-oophorectomy

the surgical term for removal of both the right and left fallopian tubes and ovaries.

The staging system is based on the findings at the time of surgery. Table 4 gives the staging system based on the International Federation of Gynecologic Oncologists (FIGO).

Total hysterectomy

removal of the uterus and cervix.

16. What is the "grade" of a cancer? Is it the same thing as the "stage"?

The *grade* is not the same thing as the *stage* of a cancer. Staging is a way of describing the location and spread of cancer. The staging system for ovarian cancer requires surgery to determine the extent of disease. The grade of cancer, on the other hand, is a way of describing the cells themselves in comparison to normal cells—a means of saying just *how* abnormal an abnormal cell appears.

Table 4 describes the staging system in detail. In general, stage I disease is limited to the ovary; stage II cancer will have spread from the ovary to other pelvic organs; stage III cancer has spread to abdominal surfaces, lymph nodes, and intestinal surfaces; and stage IV cancer will have spread to the liver or the lungs or to other distant places. The staging system serves several purposes: first, it provides a standard language so that all of the people involved in treatment of ovarian cancer, from the surgeon to the medical oncologist to the nurses, can understand the extent of disease when a woman presents with ovarian cancer. Second, it is used to decide what kind of treatment is used. Finally, it's used when we try to determine the chances that you may have in beating the cancer (your prognosis).

The grade of a cancer, on the other hand, tells us something quite different. As mentioned in Question 12, the degree of cellular change, or atypia, is an important factor in determining normal from abnormal cells. Pathologists use a scoring system to determine how greatly these cells differ from their normal counterparts; that's termed the **grade**. In this system, grade I cancers are very similar to normal tissue and are called **well-differentiated**. As cancers look increasingly abnormal, their grade gets higher. Thus, grade II cancers are **moderately differentiated**; grade III cancers are **poorly differentiated**; and grade IV cancers,

Grade

a pathologist's term that defines how abnormal a cell is under the microscope.

Well-differentiated

a pathologist's term to describe cellular changes of a cancer cell; this describes cells that meet criteria for cancer but still maintain a resemblance to normal cells.

Moderately differentiated

cells that do not resemble the normal appearance, but are still recognizable as related to their normal counterpart.

Poorly differentiated

cells that bear no resemblance to their normal counterpart.

which bear no resemblance to normal tissue, are
undifferentiated.

In some cancers, including ovarian cancer, the grade
can be used to predict how well your cancer will
respond to chemotherapy. Grade I tumors are slow-
growing and are not as responsive to chemotherapy,
but grade III tumors usually respond well because they
are much more active and dividing.

17. What is my prognosis, and how is it determined?

A **prognosis** is an assessment of how a person diagnosed with a specific disease is likely to do and gives
an estimate of the likelihood of cure or long-term survival. It is based on the information we have learned
over the years about how women with the various
stages and grades of ovarian cancer do over time. It is
not something that is carved in stone; cancer patients
with poor prognoses (i.e., the dreaded statement, "You
have six months to live") have been known to do far
better than predicted, with some surviving years, even
decades, longer than forecast by their prognoses. Every
patient is different, and your response to a particular
form of treatment may be better or worse than average,
so take the prognosis with a grain of salt.

The prognosis of patients with ovarian cancer depends
on a variety of factors. Some important factors that
have an impact on prognosis are (1) the type of cancer
as determined through the microscope; (2) the stage of
ovarian cancer; (3) whether all visible cancer was
removed at surgery (or **debulking**); (4) the size of any

Risk Factors, Diagnosis, and Staging

Undifferentiated
cells that bear no
resemblance at all to
normal cells.

*In some can-
cers, including
ovarian can-
cer, the grade
can be used to
predict how
well your
cancer will
respond to
chemotherapy.*

Prognosis
an estimate of the
outlook following the
diagnosis of a disease
such as cancer.

*The prognosis
is not some-
thing that is
carved in
stone.*

Debulking
the process of
removing cancer
from your body.

disease left after the initial surgery; and (5) your over-all medical condition and age.

The prognosis is generally good for stage I ovarian cancer. However, most patients will require additional treatment in the form of chemotherapy after surgery.

Chemotherapy is highly effective in treating ovarian cancer, and combined surgery and chemotherapy is associated with a good prognosis and a high cure rate for early stage I disease.

For more advanced stages, the prognosis will depend on the size and volume of disease that is left after ini-tial debulking. The best surgical result after the initial surgery is to leave no visible disease at the end of debulking (otherwise known as a **complete resection**). Patients with no visible remaining (residual) disease tend to have a prognosis and overall survival better than that of patients whose disease cannot be com-pletely removed (otherwise called **suboptimal debulk-ing**). If visible residual disease cannot be completely removed, it is best to leave behind the smallest amount of disease. That's usually defined as less than one cen-timeter in diameter (**optimal debulking**).

Sometimes in advanced ovarian cancer, a tumor larger than one centimeter may be located in close proximity to vital structures, such that attempts to completely remove it would cause significant injury and/or lead to permanent disfigurement or disability. In such cases, surgeons would still require chemotherapy to fight the disease left behind.

Complete resection

removal of all visible tumor in the abdomen and pelvis.

Suboptimal debulking

residual disease greater than 1 cm in diameter upon completion of surgery.

18. How does ovarian cancer spread? Does it usually spread to particular locations?

The most dangerous type of ovarian cancer—or any cancer—is cancer that has metastasized, or spread to another part of the body. The danger lies in the fact that once cancer metastasizes, it can go just about anywhere and start growing new tumors. Like other cancers, ovarian cancer that metastasizes can show up in the lungs, liver, or even the brain. However, for reasons not fully understood, this cancer seems to "prefer" the environment of the abdomen and pelvis and will most often grow and spread in these areas, even when it recurs.

Ovarian cancer can spread (metastasize) in one of three ways. In local extension, the cancer can spread locally, either by growing directly on the surface of adjacent tissue (**direct extension**) or by growing through the surface of the **peritoneum**, the inner lining of your abdomen. When it spreads by such direct extension, the cancer attaches and then spreads to the fallopian tube, uterus, bladder, peritoneum, or rectal surface. This is a common way for locally advanced disease to spread. The other way is by spreading along the peritoneum. Ovarian cancer can shed from its original site in the ovary and land anywhere on the lining of the pelvic or abdominal peritoneum, where it can form new tumor nodules covering the lining of the pelvis or the lining of the abdomen or even replacing the omentum (the normal fatty structure that drapes between the stomach and transverse colon). This is a very common site in which to find advanced ovarian cancer. When the omentum is replaced with tumor, it is commonly described as an **omental cake**.

Another path for metastasis lies through the **lymphatic channels**. Lymphatic channels form a complex

For reasons not fully understood, this cancer seems to "prefer" the environment of the abdomen and pelvis and will most often grow and spread in these areas, even when it recurs.

Direct extension

the process by which cancer extends into local and surrounding tissue.

Omental cake

tumor involvement of the omentum that results in the formation of a large mass.

Lymphatic channels

vessels through which lymph fluid travels; part of the lymphatic system.

and extensive network of channels found throughout the body. They function to drain the body of waste. Ovarian carcinoma can spread through the lymph nodes of the pelvis into the periaortic area and occasionally can even spread to lymph nodes in the chest and neck region. Approximately 20% of apparent early ovarian cancer may have disease spread outside the ovary, particularly in lymph nodes. With advanced ovarian cancer, the lymph nodes may be involved in as many as 60% of patients.

Metastasis can also take place through the bloodstream. When cancer invades into blood vessels, it can travel throughout the body, a process called **hematogenous dissemination**. It is through the bloodstream that ovarian cancer spreads to the lung, liver, or brain.

Hematogenous dissemination

a process of spread by which cancer travels through the bloodstream.

19. What sort of doctor should I consult? Should I get a second opinion? Could consulting another doctor affect my treatment or prognosis?

Choosing your doctor is ultimately a decision that can affect your outcome and your survival.

Choosing your doctor is ultimately a decision that can affect your outcome and your survival. Your primary physician probably handled matters through your initial diagnosis, and indeed may be a good person to assist you throughout your treatment. However, even if he or she is a gynecologist, your primary physician probably is not a specialist in treating ovarian cancer and therefore cannot be expected to be up to date on the latest information about this disease. Moreover, you are going to need surgery to remove the cancer, and that's something your primary physician cannot provide—but a gynecologic oncologist can. Thus, your outcome and chances of survival may be improved if you request from the beginning that a gynecologic oncologist be involved in your care, either as your primary surgeon or as a standby assistant surgeon. If you're diagnosed with ovarian cancer by your primary physician, please seek consultation with a gynecologic oncologist as soon as possible.

You could also request a referral to a gynecologic oncologist to obtain a second opinion if you wish to be absolutely certain about the nature of your illness or the type of cancer and its treatment options. A second opinion is always reasonable. In general, a second opinion is a good idea if surgery has been recommended, as the type and extent of the surgical procedure can affect overall treatment recommendations and may even alter your prognosis. Women who have all their cancer removed (complete resection) or have all but less than 1 centimeter of disease removed (optimal debulking) tend to fare better than do women whose cancer cannot be removed for technical reasons (suboptimal debulking). In general, a qualified gynecological oncologist, not a general surgeon or gynecologist, should perform any surgery for ovarian cancer.

A second opinion is a good idea if surgery has been recommended.

When it comes to chemotherapy, a second opinion is equally reasonable if you are interested in a **clinical trial** (discussed in Question 40) or a more aggressive approach beyond what is done routinely. Ongoing research is trying to improve on the results of standard treatment, and you should explore such research if you are interested. If a cancer comes back (recurs), a second opinion is very reasonable in order to explore clinical trials and the different ways to treat recurrent disease.

Andrea's comment:

I think the decision to go for a second opinion depends on how you feel about your first opinion. Consulting with a gynecological oncologic surgeon is imperative, as these doctors will have more experience with this specific, and fairly rare, disease. My insurance plan covered the cost of second opinions, and we consulted with three surgeons before deciding. All three surgeons came highly recommended by my gynecologist, my fertility specialist, a friend, and an internist. It was a matter of finding someone, along with a facility, with which both my husband and I felt comfortable and confident. I think getting too many opinions can be confusing and time-consuming, but we found the process helpful in that I felt that we had explored different doctors and approaches and found the one that was right for us.

My surgeon, Dr. Barakat, and my oncologists, first Dr. Soignet and now Dr. Dizon, have been instrumental in keeping me alive and well. We rely on the surgeon and oncologist to provide us with information and options and to make recommendations that I must take the responsibility of accepting, or questioning. I've always felt that we work as a team, although at times it's been tempting to look on the doctor as the source of salvation. But they're only human, too, doing the best of their ability, and it is of the utmost importance to build a relationship of honesty, trust, and understanding.

Whether you see one doctor or more, take someone with you who can take notes while you listen. It can be hard to take it all in at once, and it was reassuring to have someone there who could not only be a second pair of ears but provide the emotional support that comes with the presence of a trusted human being.

At some point you may find, as I did, that I was quite comfortable meeting with the doctor on my own. But it's always been important that my husband come not only in times of great need (such as when deciding on a course of treatment) but also to accompany me so that we have the experience of sharing both the decision making and the coping. This prevented me from trying to protect him from my health situation, as when I tried to do so and found myself not only not protecting him but isolating myself.

PART THREE

Treatment of Ovarian Cancer

Who is involved in my treatment?

What will the surgeon do?

Does everyone with ovarian cancer
need chemotherapy?

More ...

20. How do I decide on where to be treated?

Deciding where to obtain treatment is a very personal issue, and your comfort with your treating physician should guide you. Your relationship with your oncologist is going to be one of the most important relationships you have; for that reason, it must be based in trust and honesty. If you do not feel comfortable asking questions or you feel that your oncologist is not taking you seriously, you should find a new provider. Just as important is that your oncologist be accessible. Chemotherapy causes side effects that can require frequent visits to your doctor's office or may require you to go into a hospital. The distance you have to travel should also be a factor to consider. The worst situation is to feel sick but helpless because you live too far away.

21. Who's involved in my treatment?

It's important for you to be treated with a team of specialists that should include a medical oncologist, a surgical oncologist (preferably one who specializes in gynecologic oncology; see Question 22), a radiation oncologist, and a pathologist. The pathologist is important because this person will confirm your cancer diagnosis and help to stage (define the extent of) the disease.

For women with ovarian cancer, the gynecological oncologist may take on a double role as both surgical and medical oncologist. For others, the surgeon and the medical oncologist will work closely together. The radiation oncologist is a specialist in the use of radiation to treat cancer; although it has a limited role in women newly diagnosed, radiation may become important in women with recurrent cancer.

In addition to these physician specialists, it's important to have access to the supporting staff in the office, including but not limited to the oncology nurses, social workers, and clinical therapists who can help you and your loved ones to adjust to often difficult situations.

Andrea's comment:

Assembling a medical team and support network is crucially important. Healing takes place on many levels, known and unknown, and I think that one step toward health is choosing and having confidence in your medical team. Another is realizing and accepting the responsibility that you have as part of that team. Ultimately, the patient is the one to make the decisions and, in my case, I rely on the doctors to present options to work with. Fighting cancer is a Herculean task, and you want your support staff to be the best you can find. Don't give up until you find people with whom you can work, from whom you can learn, and in whom you can have confidence.

Sometimes it's helpful to enlist the opinion of family and friends, and some of the most positive feedback I heard was from someone who initially told me to know that I deserved to get the best care and not to be afraid to ask for it. Being sick at times made me feel very vulnerable and dependent, and I am thankful that I was always reminded that I was an integral part of the medical team: It made me feel more confident and in control of a situation that was unknowable, and chaotic. And I learned a lot when a friend prayed with me before a major surgery, asking God to guide the surgeon's hands.

Treatment of Ovarian Cancer

SURGERY

22. Who should do my surgery?

If a diagnosis of ovarian cancer is suspected or if the possibility of ovarian cancer is present, surgery is best performed by a **gynecologic oncologist**. Gynecologic oncologists are physicians who have completed a full training in general obstetrics and gynecology and have received additional specialized training in gynecologic oncology (usually 2–4 years).

Surgery for ovarian cancer is best performed where the appropriate operation can be conducted and resection of advanced disease can be as complete as possible. Unfortunately, many patients with ovarian cancer continue to have their surgery performed by non–oncologic surgeons; this results in an incomplete operation or a less aggressive attempt at resection. In such situations, a patient may require additional surgery in order to stage the disease completely or to resect advanced disease.

23. What will the surgeon do?

The first things that the surgeon will do are to study your medical history; perform a thorough examination, including a pelvic examination; and review any radiology studies. If the history review and examination suggest ovarian cancer, your surgeon will recommend surgery. The goals of surgery are to remove the primary cancer, to determine whether the cancer has spread, and to attempt to remove the spread of cancer as best as possible.

Surgery for Apparently Early Disease

If radiology exams indicate that you have localized or early ovarian cancer (generally meaning the disease is only contained in your pelvis), the surgeon will remove

Gynecological oncologist

a specialist in the treatment of cancer of the female reproductive system.

both your tubes and ovaries and your uterus. That's described as **a total abdominal hysterectomy and bilateral salpingo-oophorectomy**. In addition, your surgeon will take samples from any areas of possible tumor spread as part of the staging procedure. That would mean taking the lymph nodes from both sides of your pelvis and around the aorta, removal of the omentum, and obtaining tissue around your abdomen and pelvis (known as **peritoneal biopsies**) and washings to exclude cancer spread. If disease is present in your abdomen at the time of surgery, the goal of surgery would be to debulk or resect as much as possible, leaving the smallest possible amount of visible disease.

Advanced Disease

When ovarian cancer is advanced or widespread, more extensive surgery is usually needed, and you would likely undergo radical debulking. It is important to know that the description that follows applies only to selected patients with advanced bulky disease; it is not what early-stage ovarian cancer patients undergo. However, it provides ample reason for a newly diagnosed patient to avoid delaying treatment.

Debulking usually requires a resection of the uterus, both tubes and ovaries, possibly the rectum, and part of the large colon. If that were the case, you might require a segment of bowel pulled through your abdomen so that stool can drain (a **colostomy**). This intestinal diversion is usually temporary and may be reversed by another operation at a later date.

Colostomy
segment of bowel that is pulled through your skin.

Occasionally, segments of small intestine have to be removed. The lining of the abdomen may have implants on it, and these are also removed. Occasionally, the lining of the diaphragm also will have to be removed.

Less frequently, patients may have advanced disease involving their liver or gallbladder; in such cases, resection of these areas may become necessary. The spleen is another organ that occasionally can be involved in ovarian cancer. It is not uncommon for women to undergo a splenectomy in order to remove disease that may be involving the spleen. Occasionally, the appendix is removed as part of ovarian cancer surgery. The overall intent is to remove completely all visible sites of disease, leaving the abdomen and pelvis with the smallest amount of residual tumor.

The overall intent is to remove completely all visible sites of disease.

24. Must the surgeon remove both ovaries if I am diagnosed with ovarian cancer?

Most ovarian cancer patients are postmenopausal, so concerns about fertility are irrelevant in the majority of cases. Some patients, however, are diagnosed before menopause, and a certain proportion of them, like Andrea, are concerned about maintaining their ability to have children in the future. If you have completed your family and have no desire to remain fertile, the standard of care is to remove both your ovaries and tubes and your uterus and to perform a staging operation. This has been the traditional surgical method of treating ovarian cancer, and it is the most likely method to prevent future recurrence. However, if you strongly desire to preserve your ability to have children and have no obvious spread of cancer outside your ovary, it may possible to retain your uterus and the uninvolved tube but proceed with a full staging operation. In that procedure, the uterus and the uninvolved tube and ovary are left intact and are not removed, which would allow a woman to have children in the future. Yet even in the case of fertility-sparing surgery, the operation should still include a complete staging, which would include removal of the lymph nodes and the omentum and obtaining the peritoneal biopsies.

This conservative surgery for ovarian cancer is best reserved for young women whose disease is surgically staged as stage I, with no obvious spread of cancer outside the pelvis. The drawback to such surgery is that the risk of recurrence is considerably higher, as there is no way of knowing whether the *apparently* unaffected ovary and tubule, and the uterus, do not contain microscopic cancer deposits. Thus, a woman who chooses the conservative surgery must be alert to signs and symptoms of cancer recurrence.

Andrea's comment:

Maintaining fertility is not something most ovarian cancer patients must worry about, but it was a major concern for my husband and me. We had been married for only 1 1/2 years when I was diagnosed. We had to weigh the benefits of waiting to have surgery until eggs could be extracted or to see whether it was possible to retain an ovary against immediate and extensive surgery. One surgeon I consulted with asked if I wanted to wait a month in order to extract eggs (which we didn't, as we felt time was of the essence and wanted surgery as soon as possible); one explained to us that, given his experience with the disease and the factor of my age (39), he could only really advise removing both ovaries. My husband encouraged me to see another doctor, who said that he could see a possibility of keeping an ovary and the uterus intact if I was in early stage. This was one factor informing my choice of surgeon. However, owing to the spread of the disease, I had a full hysterectomy.

It took me a long time to mourn the loss of fertility. This has been hard on us as a couple because we so greatly wanted children. We have talked about adoption but have decided for the time being to leave it be. Time has helped us to accept these changes and to look forward instead of looking back to what could have been. Psychotherapy, both individually and in couples counseling, has helped us. But it remains poignant to remember what was lost.

CHEMOTHERAPY

25. Does everyone with ovarian cancer need chemotherapy?

Chemotherapy is recommended for every patient with ovarian cancer except those with stage IA, grade 1, or grade 2 tumors. Grade 3 cancers, even at the earliest stages, are usually treated with chemotherapy. Recently reported data based on two large trials in women with early-stage disease suggested that the addition of chemotherapy to surgery improves overall survival by 8% and improves the chances of not having it come back by 11%, compared to surgery alone.

On the basis of ongoing studies of early-stage cancers, it may be enough to receive three cycles of chemotherapy, but we are awaiting the results of a recently completed national clinical trial. For women with advanced disease, the standard recommendation is for six cycles of platinum-based chemotherapy.

26. What kind of chemotherapy is used to treat ovarian cancer?

Landmark clinical trials have established that standard treatment of epithelial ovarian cancer uses a taxane-platinum combination. These drugs are described further below.

Platinum agents (carboplatin and cisplatin) are the drugs most active in treating ovarian cancer; they work by creating breaks in the DNA, leading eventually to cell death. Although active against cancer cells, they also affect normally dividing cells, which accounts for some of their side effects. Cisplatin was used more commonly in the past, but it has significant side effects, including nausea and vomiting, potential hearing loss, kidney injury, and permanent nerve damage. Fortunately, we have learned through clinical trials that a very close cousin to cisplatin—carboplatin—is just as effective. In addition, carboplatin is less likely to injure the kidneys and nerves. Its major toxicity lies in decreasing your blood counts, which can make you prone to infection. Some nausea is associated with carboplatin but, fortunately, your physician can prescribe chemotherapy-specific antinausea drugs, such as Emend, Kytril, Anzemet, and Zofran, to make this less of a problem.

Taxanes (paclitaxel, docetaxel) work by blocking microtubules (tiny structures found in nearly all cells), thereby interrupting cells as they divide. Paclitaxel was the drug initially studied in clinical trials involving ovarian cancer patients. It is given over 24 hours if combined with cisplatin or as a 3-hour infusion when given with carboplatin, which is the more common chemotherapy program used. Recently, a large European study confirmed that docetaxel is equivalent to paclitaxel, but has fewer long-term side effects than paclitaxel.

The major side effects of paclitaxel are a total hair loss, with the most dramatic loss occurring after the first treatment, as well as numbness, tingling, or both, usually affecting the hands and feet. That sensation is usually reversible after paclitaxel is stopped. In addition, paclitaxel can cause a **hypersensitivity reaction** (your body reacting to what it thinks is a foreign substance) while the drug is being infused into your system. The reaction usually occurs during the start of the infusion and can occur during any of your treatments. It can be characterized by many types of symptoms: flushing, shortness of breath, chest pressure, chest or back pain, or rash. It can usually be managed by stopping the infusion and giving you an extra dose of antihistamines. Once the reaction subsides, paclitaxel can be restarted. This is because the reaction is caused not by paclitaxel itself but by the molecule with which it is mixed to allow it to be absorbed better into your bloodstream. Your body may react to this other substance (called a **cremaphore**) by releasing histamines that causes the reaction. Once your body releases all its histamine, the infusion can be restarted.

Cremaphore

a molecule to which drugs are attached to increase the drug's delivery into your body.

Docetaxel, on the other hand, does not cause the same degree of numbness or tingling, although it does cause hair loss. Its major side effect is decreased blood counts, which can be treated with medications that boost blood cell production.

27. What is neoadjuvant treatment?

Neoadjuvant treatment

treatment given before surgery.

The term **neoadjuvant treatment** refers to chemotherapy given before surgery instead of after. It is used sometimes when your surgeon thinks that you have a large tumor burden that can't be completely removed, or when a patient's overall condition makes surgery highly risky. This approach aims to decrease the volume of cancer so as to improve the chances of optimal debulking (resection, or removal). Studies have shown that this approach is not any less successful than surgery followed by chemotherapy.

28. How is chemotherapy administered?

The standard chemotherapy program for ovarian cancer does not require you to stay in the hospital. Your doctor will ask you to take a special medication called **dexamethasone**, the night before and the morning of your treatment. This medication is a **steroid** that is used to decrease your risk of running into trouble with a hypersensitivity reaction to paclitaxel. Both carboplatin and paclitaxel are given in one of your veins, and it usually takes 6 hours to complete. Paclitaxel is given over 3 hours and, before beginning the treatment, patients usually receive premedication with an **antihistamine** and an antinausea medication. Sometimes another dose of steroid is given, but this is up to the discretion of your physician. Carboplatin is administered over an hour. You should not require hospitalization at all for this treatment. If cisplatin is used with paclitaxel, patients are generally hospitalized, as it takes 24 hours to administer paclitaxel when used with cisplatin.

Antihistamine

to block the release of histamines, which are often associated with allergic reactions.

29. Does chemotherapy cause any long-term side effects?

Paclitaxel can cause numbness and tingling, usually felt mostly in your hands and feet (also termed **sensory neuropathy**). This can be expected to go away, albeit slowly, and it may take up to a year from the time you end treatment before your numbness goes away completely. If you experience this symptom, talk to your doctor or nurse, as they may have some suggestions to alleviate it. Hair loss is temporary, however, and you should start to notice your hair coming back within 3 months from the end of treatment. Your tiredness will probably get worse as you approach the end of your treatment (i.e., the fifth and sixth treatments); likely

Sensory neuropathy

numbness and tingling, usually involving the hands and feet.

you won't have the same energy level that you had prior to treatment. This may last for a couple of months, but then you should slowly start to feel like yourself once it is completed.

You shouldn't expect any residual side effects from carboplatin. Rarely, it can cause worsening of hearing loss, particularly in older patients and those with a baseline hearing loss. If you already have hearing loss, it must be followed (monitored) while you are being treated.

TREATMENT OF NONEPITHELIAL OVARIAN CANCER

30. When do germ-cell tumors require chemotherapy?

In women diagnosed with early-stage disease, postsurgical treatment using chemotherapy is usually reserved for those with any of the following types of tumors: embryonal carcinomas, endodermal sinus tumors, or mixed germ-cell tumors. Women with these types of tumors are at a high risk of relapse, so chemotherapy is given after surgery in the hope that the drugs will destroy any tumor cells that might remain after surgery and thus prevent recurrence. Chemotherapy is also given in women who have advanced germ-cell tumors or in whom tumors have returned.

The general-treatment uses drugs different from those used for epithelial cancers. The most common regimen (program or schedule) is bleomycin, etoposide, and cisplatin (BEP). It has been shown to be very active in the treatment of germ-cell cancers.

However, this regimen is not without risks, and the potential benefit of treatment has to be weighed against the side effects of the treatment. Because women with germ-cell tumors are typically young when they are diagnosed, these considerations should not be taken lightly.

The major side effects that need to be considered are damage from bleomycin to your lungs, which can happen during or after treatment and can lead to scarring (or **pulmonary fibrosis**); damage from cisplatin to your nerves and kidneys, which can be permanent; and a risk (although rare) from etoposide of causing leukemia later in life.

Pulmonary fibrosis
scarring of the lung tissue, which is generally not reversible.

More than 90% of patients with germ-cell tumors will be cured after the BEP program. The number of treatments is generally three or four cycles given every 3 weeks, although your physician may recommend more if your disease has spread or if treatment has to be changed due to side effects that occur while you're on BEP.

31. Do all types of sex cord–stromal tumors require chemotherapy?

No, not all sex cord or stromal tumors require chemotherapy. Many of these tumors will require only surgery, but it's important that surgical staging be complete, particularly in women who want to keep their fertility.

Early-stage granulosa-cell tumors do not warrant treatment after surgery. Even for women with advanced disease, the benefit of postoperative treatment with radiation, chemotherapy, or hormones is not completely clear. In such a case, your oncologist may recommend no further treatment except regular visits to the office every 3 to 4 months.

Even when disease recurs, surgery is the preferred choice of treatment. Your oncologist may offer chemotherapy, but this decision is an individual choice based on how much cancer was found, the length of time before the cancer came back, and how strong you are at the time of the recurrence. If chemotherapy becomes necessary, the regimen of choice is BEP. The optimal management for women with recurrent or incompletely resected disease has not been established.

32. Is chemotherapy ever recommended for borderline tumors?

Chemotherapy has no standard role in treating borderline tumors. The major treatment is surgical. If the entire tumor is removed, particularly if it is found at an early stage, women with these tumors are generally cured. Even if the disease has spread outside your pelvis, all attempts at removing all visible disease afford the best chance of survival; chemotherapy may or may not be recommended. In general, chemotherapy is reserved for tumors that were incompletely removed surgically or else are found through the microscope to be invasive (which can signify a more aggressive tendency to the borderline tumor, or even actual cancer). If chemotherapy is warranted, the tumor is treated with carboplatin and paclitaxel, just as for ovarian cancer.

33. Are any tumor markers associated with these non-epithelial types of ovarian tumors?

CA-125 results are sometimes increased in women with borderline tumors.

For the germ-cell tumors, two types of proteins are often elevated. These are the human chorionic gonadotropin (or the hCG) and alpha-feto protein (AFP). The hCG is what is tested in a pregnancy test, but in this situation it is used to monitor the activity of both nongestational choriocarcinomas and dysgerminomas to treatment. The AFP is a tumor marker as well, and is elevated in endodermal sinus tumors, immature teratoma, and the embryonal carcinomas.

The sex cord–stromal tumors can cause increased estrogen and progesterone levels but do not usually have a tumor marker. One exception is the granulosa-cell tumor, which secretes a protein known as inhibin. Other useful markers may include LDH and CA-125.

34. What happens if the CA-125 result isn't normal during chemotherapy?

The CA-125 reading should decrease gradually with treatment. Ideally, it should be normal after the third treatment, although this may depend on how high the CA-125 result was when you started treatment. If it is going down slowly, your doctor may recommend additional cycles of treatment, usually up to eight cycles. If the number flattens out or starts to rise, it may indicate that your cancer is not responding to the treatment. It is important that a repeat evaluation be performed in that situation, usually with a CT (computed tomography) scan. Signs signaling that the disease isn't responding call for a change in plan, as more of the same treatment is unlikely to help you.

If your disease stops responding to up-front treatment, your doctor may describe your cancer as "primary platinum-refractory." In women with platinum-refractory disease, the cancer is not curable. Instead, the goal of further therapy becomes one of control. This approach is similar to that taken for women with recurrent ovarian cancer, particularly if the cancer comes back in a short time (within 3 months of stopping treatment). The management (handling) of recurrent and refractory cancers is discussed later in this book (see Part Six).

35. Does radiation play a role?

Although it's not considered a standard treatment for ovarian cancer, radiation is an effective means of treatment. It has fallen out of favor as adjuvant treatment (i.e., after surgery) because chemotherapy has been shown to be an effective means of therapy. When used after initial surgery, radiation is directed against the entire abdomen; this carries a risk of complications to your bowel and kidneys. Therefore, it's usually reserved for treatment of recurrent tumors, particularly in situations in which an isolated recurrence can be encompassed in one radiation field.

POSTREMISSION TREATMENT
36. What is second-look surgery?

After initial surgery and an initial course of chemotherapy, ovarian cancer in many patients will be considered in remission as the result of physical examination, tumor marker assay, and imaging tests. In other words, physical examination will reveal no evidence of disease, the CA-125 results will be normal, and a CT (computed tomography) scan of the abdomen and pelvis will be negative. This is described as **clinical complete remission**. Unfortunately, especially in women with stage III and stage IV disease, a clinical remission may not mean a **pathologic remission**. That is, although the clinical picture appears to show no evidence of cancer, by looking inside your abdomen and taking biopsies from areas of usual tumor persistence, your oncologist may find persistent disease. Thus, oncologists sometimes perform what is called a "second-look" surgery.

The second-look operation for ovarian cancer has been performed for several decades. By definition, a second-look operation is a surgical procedure to evaluate the status of your cancer after up-front chemotherapy and whether you appear to be free of cancer after such surgery and chemotherapy. The aim of a second-look is to obtain multiple biopsies from your abdomen and pelvis and to obtain washings in order to evaluate the presence of any residual cancer after primary surgery and chemotherapy.

In many cases, this operation can be performed by a camera-directed, minimally invasive procedure called a **laparoscopy**, although occasionally a more extensive abdominal incision will be made. The second-look operation can provide important information, particularly by telling both you and your physician how successful chemotherapy was according to the presence or

---

Treatment of Ovarian Cancer

Clinical complete remission

a normal physical exam, tumor marker, and radiology tests following the completion of treatment for cancer.

Pathological remission

the finding of no residual cancer at the end of primary treatment for cancer; only diagnosed in a second surgical procedure.

Laparoscopy

camera-directed surgery done without creating a large incision into the abdomen.

absence of cancer. If your oncologist identifies visible residual disease in the process, it may be resected (removed), and that may be helpful to you. Additional treatment can be planned after a second-look operation, such as abdominally directed treatment through an **intraperitoneal port**.

The available data suggest that approximately 50% of women with disease that appears to be in clinical remission will have no evidence of cancer at second look. Owing to the lack of sufficient noninvasive diagnostics tools, the second-look operation has remained the only way to tell clearly whether your disease is in complete remission pathologically. Nevertheless, many institutions do not routinely use second-look surgery because of the uncertainty about how beneficial it might be.

37. What is intraperitoneal chemotherapy?

Intraperitoneal (IP) chemotherapy, otherwise known as a **belly wash**, is a way of infusing chemical agents (drugs) directly into your abdomen (the peritoneal cavity). The IP route requires placement of a temporary catheter in your abdomen that's connected to a small plastic container (a **reservoir**) positioned underneath the skin, usually right on top of your lower rib cage. The reservoir can be accessed with a needle through the skin, which allows drugs to be given directly into your abdomen. The agents are allowed to spread throughout the peritoneal cavity (hence the term "belly wash") and eventually are absorbed through the abdominal lining over the next 1 to 2 days. This

Intraperitoneal port

a surgically placed device inserted under the skin and into the abdomen, which allows directed treatment into the abdomen.

Intraperitoneal

into the abdomen.

Belly wash

common term for an intraperitoneal treatment.

Reservoir

a receptacle that holds fluid.

method of administering chemotherapy is attractive for patients with ovarian cancer because this disease tends to spread through the lining of the abdomen and, in many cases, stays in the peritoneal cavity. The goal of this directed approach is to target any possible remaining ovarian cancer cells and destroy them in the hope of prolonging a disease-free survival and overall survival.

The goal of this directed approach is to target any possible remaining ovarian cancer cells and destroy them in the hope of prolonging a disease-free survival and overall survival.

IP chemotherapy has been evaluated as part of the up-front treatment in women with Stage III ovarian cancer who have no or little disease after surgery (i.e., those who were optimally debulked). The results of three randomized trials showed that a combination of intravenous and IP chemotherapy is associated with a survival benefit over standard intravenous treatment. However, the toxicity of the treatment has made use of IP therapy difficult. Therefore, the combination continues to be evaluated in clinical trials to define a regimen that is safer and better tolerated.

IP therapy has also been used in consolidation (see Question 38), although it has not been tested in randomized trials. This appears to work best for patients who have disease that can be seen only under a microscope or those who have a very-small-volume disease. Often, the limitation on whether a woman can get IP therapy is the amount of scarring in her abdomen (**adhesions**). The therapy should be used only in patients who have minimal or no intra-abdominal adhesions, because such scarring will interfere with the way the drug spreads throughout the belly. If you have a lot of adhesions, the agents will not reach all parts of the peritoneum and may not get into the areas where cancer cells live.

Adhesions

scarring within the abdominal cavity that commonly occurs after surgery.

The IP catheter and reservoir are removed after the treatment is completed. This generally does not require a large surgery and is often performed in an outpatient setting under local anesthesia without much difficulty or complications. The IP catheter and reservoir, like any other foreign device in humans, carry a small risk of infection or malfunction, and occasionally the catheter has to be removed due to either malfunction or infection.

The main side effects during the treatment are feeling distended or cramping during administration of the chemotherapeutic agent. However, the drug can be absorbed into your bloodstream, and this can cause side effects.

38. What does consolidation mean?

When used in the treatment of ovarian cancer, **consolidation** refers to additional treatment offered to women who, after completing surgery and chemotherapy, have no cancer detectable by examination, radiology studies, or CA-125. The goal of this extra treatment, it's hoped, is to increase the odds that the cancer will not come back (recur). At some medical centers, this extra treatment may consist of further chemotherapy administered by vein; at other select centers, an intraperitoneal approach is used, as described in the preceding question (Question 37).

The other option for consolidation is to use more chemotherapy by vein without a second-look operation, as long as your disease meets the criteria that define a clinical remission: a normal physical examination result, a normal CA-125 reading, and a normal CT scan.

If you're interested in these options, it's best to discuss them with your oncologist. The choice of consolidation is very center- and physician-dependent because never has a randomized trial (test with patients) definitively proved that consolidation translated into an improved survival. A recently completed randomized trial has shown that extending paclitaxel treatment as a monthly treatment for a year results in a longer duration without your cancer progressing, compared to a regimen of paclitaxel given monthly for 3 months. The study was terminated early due to this positive result, but the question of whether this translates into your surviving in the long-term remains unknown.

OTHER THERAPIES

39. What is a vaccine?

When we were kids, we routinely received a series of shots to protect us from infections. Those were **vaccines**. However, the role of vaccines in the fight against ovarian cancer is an area of active research.

As they relate to cancer treatment, vaccines are a novel way of stopping cancer from spreading by teaching the body's immune system to recognize the tumor cells as foreign and kill them off. There are various preparations of vaccines: Some are based on an individual's specific tumor, others are based on common molecules found in a majority of ovarian cancers, and still others are directed against CA-125. All are in clinical development throughout the country and are being tested in a number of ways to learn how to use them in battling ovarian cancer. All vaccines are still considered investigational, and you generally can receive them only if you are participating in a clinical trial. One vaccine,

Vaccine

a preparation that is given to induce immunity to a disease or condition.

Treatment of Ovarian Cancer

MAb B43.13 (oregovomab, Ovarex™), is currently in a phase III randomized trial across the country for women who have completed up-front treatment for Stage III or IV ovarian cancer.

40. When should I consider a clinical trial?

Participating in clinical trials (studies using patients) is always an option for women in all phases of ovarian cancer, from initial diagnosis to relapse to second remission. However, the vast majority of women turn to clinical trials only after standard therapy has failed.

There are no guidelines in place as to when a patient should participate in a clinical trial. Before you begin investigating trial options, it is important to understand the different types of studies done in cancer research, because not all trials are the same, and you need to look for one that is suited to your circumstances.

There are three basic types of clinical trials. Phase I trials are the earliest type of clinical trials. They are designed to test a new medication or treatment strategy, and often they are "first-in-human" studies involving only a small number of patients. The main purpose of these trials is to determine the best dose of a new drug or treatment to take into further development. This is done by starting at a low dose and gradually increasing it until side effects are seen. This leads us to the second goal of these early trials: to determine what kind of side effects are associated with the new treatment being tested. It's important to realize that although most phase I trials want to test whether the study drug can cause tumors to shrink, it is not the primary goal.

The vast majority of women turn to clinical trials only after standard therapy has failed.

Once a phase I trial is completed, the next step in development of a new treatment is to define how active a drug is. That's the goal of a phase II trial. Unlike phase I trials, the majority of phase II trials are conducted to target specific diseases. In general, all patients enrolled in these studies are treated with the study medication.

If a drug or treatment looks promising in a phase II trial, the next step—a phase III trial—involves comparing it against an accepted treatment in a specific disease setting. The goal is to determine whether the treatment being tested is better than the current available treatment. These are usually run as randomized trials (participating patients are assigned randomly to a treatment). Neither they nor their doctors can select the treatment they'll receive. The results of these trials usually determine the standard of care for oncologists.

For women with newly diagnosed ovarian cancer, phase II and phase III trials are available nationally, either through research centers as single-institution studies (meaning that a certain type of treatment is being studied in only one place) or as part of a cooperative group trials (meaning that patients are being offered the trial in multiple places). For women with recurrent cancers of the ovary, all three types of trials may be available. Many of the trials limit entry by the number of prior therapies, and this is decided by the physicians and scientists studying the treatment.

Often, patients who have had two or three different treatments are excluded from the trial; although exclusion is a controversial subject (no one wants to be denied a treatment that could save her life), there are some legitimate concerns that cause investigators to refuse women previously treated with other medications access to the trial. For example, many chemotherapy regimens are toxic, not just to cancer cells, but to organs such as the liver or the kidneys. If the clinical trial drug is thought to be equally or more toxic, the investigators might be concerned that women with toxicity from prior therapy could get sicker, not healthier, by participating in the trial. Fortunately, in trials of the new targeted therapies, these concerns are less significant, so women previously treated with other drugs can often be admitted into such trials. Nevertheless, this consideration is important because it may affect your options to receive standard treatments before you enter the study.

If something is being tested in a clinical trial, its benefit is still unproven.

It's important to understand that the purpose of a clinical trial is to test a theory, in this case usually a question of the effectiveness of a new treatment strategy. If something is being tested in a clinical trial, its benefit is still unproven. It's never wrong to explore clinical trial options for any stage of ovarian cancer, and remember: All of the current *standard* therapies were once unproven—they only became standard therapies because they passed through clinical trials. However, the goals of the trial should be clearly stated and understood before you make the decision (see the Appendix for more information on clinical trials).

41. Does treatment differ if I'm pregnant when diagnosed with ovarian cancer?

Most women who get ovarian cancer do so after menopause. Pregnancy-associated ovarian cancer is a rare, but devastating, diagnosis. It can occur in 1 in

12,000 to 50,000 pregnancies. Often the diagnosis is made surgically, after women present with an abnormal routine ultrasound showing a complex cyst. CT scans are not safe in pregnancy; however, if a complex cyst is found by ultrasound in a pregnant patient, then an MRI may be done.

The first step in management is surgical, as it would be if you were not pregnant. Every attempt should be made at complete surgical staging, which means that an open procedure or laparotomy must be performed.

Unfortunately the decisions are not ones made easily. If you have advanced cancer with spread around the pelvis or abdomen, then your doctors may recommend that the pregnancy be terminated so that the most aggressive treatment can be used to give you the best chance of surviving the cancer. If you are early-staged but considered at a high risk for recurrence, some may advocate delaying treatment until after the first trimester, or even after the birth of your child, while others may recommend a more aggressive course. On the other end of the spectrum, you may be considered cured after the affected ovary is removed.

If, whatever the circumstance, you decide to continue with the pregnancy, your doctors must take into account *your* life first and foremost, all the while minimizing the potential risk to the unborn child.

There's not much information to help guide the post-surgical treatment of ovarian cancer in pregnancy. What we do know is that chemotherapy isn't safe during the first trimester, when all of your baby's organs are forming. However, beyond that, it can be safely administered, although there's always the risk of side effects.

Of the chemotherapy available to treat ovarian cancer, the little data available suggest that cisplatin is safe during pregnancy. Carboplatin may also be used, although the risk for lowering of the platelets (thrombocytopenia) may make cisplatin the better choice. The data on paclitaxel is much less clear, and it's not recommended during pregnancy. In women with early stage disease, the potential benefits of chemotherapy must be weighed against the risks of treatment.

Numerous factors must be taken into account, and you, your family, your oncologist, and your obstetrician must engage in a thorough and honest discussion about the pros and cons of all your options.

42. Is there any role for complementary or alternative therapy?

Alternative therapy (medicines used in lieu of standard medical therapies) and **complementary therapy** (medicines used in conjunction with standard therapies) include a variety of herbal and food remedies, vitamins and other supplements, and traditional treatments such as acupuncture. Such therapies have become increasingly popular with the general public, and many are based upon traditional healing practices that have hundreds of years of use. Whether they actually work is difficult to know due to the lack of scientific information available on these types of treatments. Some alternative therapies are nothing more than scams taking advantage of patients' fears and longings for anything that will make the illness go away. They may do no harm—although some herbal agents can harm you—but they also do no good, so you're spending your money for no good reason. Some alternative healing practices also address some of the emotional and physiological problems that accompany cancer treatment, so using them may improve the patient's quality of life, even if it doesn't necessarily stop the cancer itself.

Many people are becoming attracted to alternative philosophies of patient care, particularly east and south Asian methods, homeopathic, and naturopathic medical systems. Yet there are so many medicines and therapies touted as the next new treatment for cancer, it's hard to know where to start. For a cancer patient anxious to find an effective treatment—or even a way to deal with unpleasant treatment side effects—the list can be bewildering, yet a recent study of cancer patients showed that as many of 80% were using or had tried such treatments in conjunction with their standard therapeutic regimens, in the hope of either enhancing the action of the regimen or reducing the side effects caused by it. Unfortunately, a large proportion of the patients in the study were taking these alternative therapies without letting their doctors know and suffering side effects as the therapies interfered with or interacted with the action of chemotherapy drugs—which is why many physicians are wary of alternative medicines. Yet part of the problem is that doctors fail to ask whether their patients are using alternative therapies, and patients don't think to tell them. So the most important point to make in any discussion of alternative therapies is: Make sure your doctor knows about them before you start using them.

Make sure your doctor knows about any alternative therapies that interest you before you start using them.

Relaxation Therapy

Although there isn't much research on the topic of alternative medicine, it's safe to assume that therapy aimed at relaxing the mind can have a positive impact on a patient fighting cancer. Relaxation therapy, including massage, yoga, or tai chi, may provide a benefit to the patient by relieving the psychological stress associated with a cancer diagnosis.

Homeopathic and Naturopathic Medicine

Homeopathic and naturopathic medicine are also examples of complete alternative medical systems. Homeopathic medicine is an unconventional Western system that is based on the principle that "like cures like," that is, that the same substance that in large doses produces the symptoms of an illness, in very minute doses cures it. Naturopathic medicine views disease as a sign that the processes by which the body naturally heals itself are out of balance and emphasizes health restoration rather than disease treatment. Naturopathic physicians employ an array of healing practices, including diet and clinical nutrition; homeopathy; acupuncture; herbal medicine; hydrotherapy (the use of water in a range of temperatures and methods of applications); spinal and soft-tissue manipulation; physical therapies involving electric currents, ultrasound, and light therapy; therapeutic counseling; and pharmacology. Regarding homeopathic and naturopathic remedies, some physicians may recommend not taking antioxidants while on chemotherapy. This is because, in theory, chemotherapy acts by causing oxidative damage to cancer cells, so antioxidants could work against the activity of chemotherapy. If you're going to use alternative medications while undergoing treatment, it's very important to review them with your oncologist to make sure none of them interfere with standard treatments.

Andrea's comment:

I consulted with an oncologist who specializes in Chinese medicine soon after I began treatment. He made the distinc-

tion of two separate phases of complimentary treatment; first, as I had chosen the course of chemotherapy, to get me through the chemo in relatively good condition, and then once the treatment was over, to find ways to strengthen, and prevent recurrence. I brought the recommended list of supplements to my oncologist, who reviewed and accepted the supplements I would take to protect my digestive tract, help with nausea, and in general help keep me strong.

The Chinese doctor also talked about my "chi" and how during abdominal surgery, according to Chinese medicine, a lot of "chi" escapes. Thinking about it this way helped me to respect my body and think about building up my life force in general and not only focusing on the specifics of what foods to eat or not to eat. Fresh air, sunshine, fresh water, good simple food, and conscious exercise (especially the Chinese exercises, such as tai chi and chi gong, although I have preferred yoga) all contribute to the healthy buildup of one's chi.

After my diagnosis, I reconnected with a childhood friend, Carrie Lindia, who is a hands-on healer and practices Reiki. I like the idea of this kind of spiritual, hands-on healing and feel it has had a powerful effect. I've learned to practice it on myself and now, after treatment, I am learning more about it.

Soon after my first chemotherapy, I met a person who would radically change the course of my response to the illness and its treatment. Gene Fairly had been practicing Zen meditation for 25 years when he was diagnosed with a deadly throat cancer. After undergoing unsuccessful, hospitalized treatments of chemotherapy and radiation, he was told that he should undergo a major surgery, which had only a limited chance of success and would result in the loss of his voice. Without this surgery, he was told he faced a prognosis of 3 months to live. He knew instinctively that he would not survive the surgery, and as a producer, editor, translator, and great communicator, he did not want to live without the power to speak. Within 6 months of up to 6 hours a day of intensive meditation, the mass was gone. Having learned and practiced new ways to harness meditation to heal, he devoted his time after his diagnosis and cure to further developing mind–body meditation techniques and teaching them to others.

When I arrived at Gene's home the first time, I was totally overwhelmed and frightened, by the shock of surgery, the specter of chemotherapy, the fear of death. With his guidance, I learned to meditate to acknowledge and dissolve my fear; to listen to cancer cells; to meditate during chemotherapy to direct the flow of medicine to the tumor sites and to protect the healthy cells; to detoxify my liver and kidneys a few days after chemo was completed; and simply to learn the grace of feeling an inner healing power. I meditated before surgery to ask my cells to be calm and be prepared for the surgeon's work, and to cooperate. I meditated to build red and white blood cells when they were low and to face my worst fears.

One might see meditation as giving a sense of control, and it did provide that. But it also imparted peace and, in peace, there's more room for healing than there is in fear. And I fully believe that the mind "does not rest above the body but is diffused through it."[1] Learning to use the power of the mind for physical, emotional, and spiritual healing affected me in a profound way. Gene always said, "If you meditate,

---

[1]Frank WW. *The Wounded Storyteller: Body, Illness, and Ethics.* Chicago: University of Chicago Press, 1995, p. 2.

you will change." I knew that to survive this illness, I needed to change.

I also briefly tried acupuncture, which I found soothing but was unable to keep up financially. However, I connected to the acupuncturist when he talked about the fatigue being on a "sub-cellular" level.

WHAT TO DO AFTER TREATMENT IS FINISHED

43. Will the CA-125 reading ever go down to zero?

No, it usually will not go down to zero. During your treatment, we will expect that the CA-125 results will **normalize**, which in most laboratories is to fall below the level of 35 mg/dL. In most women, this means a fall in their CA-125 to the single digit or teens, but in others it will be slightly higher. As long as these changes stay below 35, there is usually no need to be alarmed. Remember that the CA-125 is only one part of the follow-up. It must be taken into consideration with other factors: how you are feeling, your physical examination, and if necessary, a CT (computed tomography) scan.

44. How often should I be examined?

If, at the end of your treatment, the cancer can't be detected, either on your physical examination, by CT scan, or by your CA-125 reading, you enter routine follow-up. Most experts agree that being seen every 3 months for the first 2 years is enough. These visits should consist of a physical assessment that includes a pelvic examination and CA-125 test. In most women

The recurrence generally appears within the first two years.

who have their cancer come back, the recurrence generally appears within this time frame. After 2 years, visits can be extended. If your chemotherapy isn't being administered by your surgeon, we feel it's important to continue to follow with both your surgeon and medical oncologist at regular intervals.

45. Do I need CT scans every three months?

There is no standard recommendation on the frequency of doing repeat CT scans. If you're doing well at your visits and there doesn't appear to be a concern that your cancer has started to grow again, there's no role for a CT scan. However, if your CA-125 reading starts to rise or goes beyond the normal range or you start to experience vague symptoms, a CT scan may be recommended. In some women, the CA-125 is not a marker of their cancer, or it was normal at the time they were diagnosed. In such situations, more attention needs to be paid to the examination results and your symptoms, but it's reasonable to perform CT scans to reevaluate your disease at more frequent intervals, such as every 3 to 6 months.

46. When can I consider myself cured?

In women who are diagnosed with ovarian cancer and have a complete resection or an optimal debulking of their cancer, chemotherapy is done with the intent to cure. Unfortunately, there's no guarantee that you'll be cured. We do know that 80% of women will initially respond to treatment, but only around 30% will not have their cancer return. In clinical studies, we often use an arbitrary time point to determine "cure," and this is 5 years. Once you get past the 5-year mark, the likelihood of the cancer returning becomes lower and lower, and the chances of your living through the cancer become better and better.

47. Do I still need yearly mammograms?

We always recommend continued health maintenance examinations once patients complete treatment. This is because the risk of a second cancer is higher in patients who have already had one type of cancer. So, yes, you will still need a mammogram. Other health maintenance tests that you and your doctor should discuss are a screening colonoscopy and a bone density test (especially if you had both ovaries removed and are not on estrogen replacement, as there is an increased risk for osteoporosis).

The risk of a second cancer is higher in patients who have already had one type of cancer.

PART FOUR

Coping with Treatment and Side Effects

Will I feel terrible during treatment?

Can I work while receiving treatment?

How will treatment affect my sex life?

More ...

48. Will I feel terrible during treatment?

Although there will be several days after treatment when you will likely feel tired and may experience varying degrees of nausea, for the most part carboplatin and paclitaxel are well-tolerated. Many patients are surprised that carboplatin and paclitaxel are not so hard on their systems. In fact, it has been shown that most women experience an improvement in their ability to enjoy life while being treated, which can be unexpected, but definitely is welcome. After all, treatments should not be worse than the disease itself and when faced with a potentially chronic disease, like ovarian cancer can be, the goal is NOT to stress your system to the point you cannot tolerate subsequent treatments. In addition, with the use of other medications to control any side effects, such as laxatives for constipation and antinausea medications, we hope to get you through the treatments without significant disability.

Andrea's comment:

For me, the immediate prospect of "chemo" was terrifying, and the first time I heard the word uttered from the oncologist's mouth, I just turned my head to the wall (this was after surgery, in the hospital) and shut down. Luckily, my husband was there to listen, but I'm sure that that experience is not so uncommon, and doctors have to broach the subject more than once. The next time around, I was able to face the prospect with greater strength, and learned that with the antinausea drugs, chemo is much more manageable than it was in even the recent past. Somehow, I learned to view the chemo not as a dreaded poison but as a powerful agent in my fight, and I learned, too, to meditate during the administration and visualize it being attracted to the cancer cells like a magnet and zapping them. I also visualized the healthy cells being protected, and learned from my meditation teacher to trust that the mind knew how to direct the message.

During the actual administration of the chemo, I never felt sick, just frightened, especially the first time. A day or two after treatment, I would feel very tired and experience nausea. Taking the antinausea medications as prescribed helped me to avoid experiencing overwhelming nausea, but they did have the side effect (along with the chemo, no doubt) of causing constipation. I found out the hard way that they should be taken as preventatives and not after the train of nausea has left the station. Then, by day five, I started feeling better, with fatigue abating and getting regular again. I found it helpful to keep a diary of how I was feeling and what I was eating, what side effects I felt, so that each cycle I could review my notes and know what to expect. The first time was the most difficult for me, I think mostly because of my fear of the unknown. I also think my body learned to adapt to the treatments, and they became less of a shock, although cumulative in negatively affecting my blood counts.

On one course using a milder drug, I got by with drinking peppermint tea and candied ginger. Chinese sailors use ginger to offset seasickness, and it worked for me during my treatment with topotecan.

There's a cycle of short-term side effects, which occur pretty much a day or two after treatment and which for me were resolved fairly quickly, and there is the longer-term side effect of physical and mental fatigue and, with that, depression and isolation. During chemo, for fatigue there are blood-boosting medications available. I found that I needed to consult a therapist, once the chemo was over, to help me move through posttreatment anxiety and depression.

Probably the most disconcerting reaction I had was to the steroids I had to take in order to keep receiving the chemo without incurring an allergic reaction. The only advice I can give here is to be sure to communicate to your nurse and to your doctor—and to the hospital's psychiatry staff if need be—if you experience any extreme emotional changes. The effects of these drugs were insidious, and I jokingly referred to the effect as having "PMS on steroids." You know how you find yourself at odds with the world and then somehow remember, Oh yeah, it's that time of the month? I think I had an unusual reaction, and it was important to me to talk to the doctor about it, and we did find a drug that helped to ease the psychological distress associated with the steroid use.

49. What side effects can I expect from chemotherapy?

Common side effects on chemotherapy include nausea, tiredness, and an effect on your bone marrow, where your infection-fighting **white blood cells,** oxygen-carrying **red blood cells,** and **platelets,** which help stop bleeding, are made. It is this effect on the bone marrow that makes you prone to getting an infection and a fever (due to the lowering of the white cells, also termed **leukopenia**), tiredness (due to lowering of your red cells, or **anemia**), or even bleeding (due to decrease in the platelets, called **thrombocytopenia**).

In addition to all of these, the different chemotherapy drugs used in the treatment of ovarian cancer have other side effects. These are listed, along with the various drugs, in Table 6 on p. 12.

Andrea's comment:

You will most likely have some nausea and queasiness; I used to describe it as like the feeling one would have after eating half a cheesecake. The treatments use pretty powerful medicines, and it takes the body some time to process them. So there are two kinds of side effects: the immediate effects of digestive problems caused by the chemo and antinausea drug effects on the digestive tract, which will resolve themselves fairly quickly, and the longer-term side effects due to lowering of blood counts, which may be cumulative, such as fatigue. I had short-term nausea and short-term fatigue, and over the course of treatments, I definitely got progressively more tired. And because of the tiredness, I experienced the psychological side effects of isolation, because sometimes I was just too tired to venture out much. I think that the isolation for me has been one of the biggest hurdles to overcome.

Drink at least a liter of water or sparkling water a day if you can. Fresh air, clean water, and exercising go a long way to revive the body. I took dry "skin brush" baths (brushing your skin with a natural fiber brush while dry). This too was a way of caring for myself, which I found to be very important and comforting during chemo. Giving my body the message of love and care was a comfort to me.

And keep moving. It made sense to me that neuropathy happened more readily if the chemo was allowed to "pool" in the extremities, but this is probably an unscientific opinion.

50. Should I take special precautions while on chemotherapy?

Many people are under the impression that chemotherapy will require them to live in their homes unable to eat fresh fruit, enjoy flowers, other people, the movies, or even their own children or grand-children. Yes, chemotherapy requires some diligence in terms of monitoring your own temperature if you feel warm or suspect a fever, but a woman doesn't need to change her entire life and surroundings due to the type of chemotherapy we use for ovarian cancer. The reason that many of these precautions are taken is to avoid any risk of infection when you are most vulnerable after chemotherapy, which is when your white counts decrease (called neutropenia) and you are prone to develop infections and fever. This time at risk is variable depending on what cancer you have and the regimen being used to treat it. People undergoing treatment for leukemia or who have had a bone marrow transplant are most at risk because the periods of neutropenia are very long. Fortunately, for women being treated for ovarian cancer, this time is not long-lasting and in general lasts less than a week. Therefore, they do not need to undergo this degree of protection.

A woman doesn't need to change her entire life and surroundings due to the type of chemotherapy we use for ovarian cancer.

Andrea's comment:

When your blood counts are predictably low, it's probably best to avoid close-quartered public spaces, such as movie theaters, where you might be exposed to a lot of people sneezing and coughing. I've heard it said to avoid eating sushi, but also I've heard that you should avoid eating raw fruit and vegetables. However, I cannot see going through chemo without eating raw fruit and some easy-to-fix salads. Just wash the food carefully, and you can soak it in a large bowl of water with a capful of peroxide to kill germs.

Mouth sores can be a side effect, although more likely a later one, and I found that brushing regularly with a soft toothbrush and rinsing my mouth regularly with a "natural" mouthwash (milder than the really strong stuff) kept me free of these sores. As soon as I started to feel one, I would begin the regular rinsing, and they would go away.

As it is important to eat, it is hard to say "eat lightly" when you might not feel like eating at all, but right after treatment, when your body is trying to process the chemo, I found it helpful to eat light, nutritious foods that I could easily digest. It also helps to eat small quantities all day rather than just a few large meals. And drink water, more water, and then some more.

51. Can I take hormones for hot flashes?

Hot flashes are a particularly difficult symptom for women with ovarian cancer, particularly if they were prematurely put into menopause after their surgery. The majority of women with epithelial ovarian cancer may be candidates for estrogen therapy if they suffer from significant hot flashes or other symptoms of menopause. Still, the use of estrogen therapy may be avoided during chemotherapy. If hot flashes are a significant problem, your doctor may recommend alternatives to estrogen for treatment, such as selected antidepressants shown to be effective in controlling menopausal symptoms. If non-hormonal strategies do not appear to work, then a frank discussion must take place between you and your doctor as to the use of hormone replacement therapy.

Andrea's comment:

This is a question between you and your doctor. I didn't start HRT (hormone replacement therapy) until after my chemo treatment was finished. I pretty much went into instant menopause, which I'm sure was a shock to my system, but I didn't feel comfortable taking HRT during chemo treatment. I think everyone has different needs here and, as my hot flashes weren't too bad, I didn't suffer a lot. However, after chemo was finished, I did take estrogen for a while and now take a low-dose intravaginal pill, mainly to keep my vagina from getting too thin or too easily chafed from lack of estrogen. There's also the option of an estrogen ring that's inserted into the vagina and time-releases estrogen.

52. Should I avoid certain foods while on chemotherapy?

There's a substantial amount of information about diet and its role in healing and cancer therapy. Unfortunately, none of it has been studied to any great degree, and there aren't a lot of data to help to guide us in the role of diet in cancer care. A lot of patients have heard about avoiding refined sugar or white flour, as these may contribute to cancer. The bottom line is that no studies have linked diet to chemotherapy response or to a risk of recurrence. It is probably best to eat a variety of foods in moderation and to follow a heart-healthy diet. After all, the cancer does not define the patient. You are still the same person you were before cancer, at risk for heart disease and high blood pressure. Treat your body well by eating a balanced diet and allow yourself the time to heal.

Treat your body well by eating a balanced diet and allow yourself the time to heal.

53. Will I be able to tolerate treatment as I get older?

Treating older patients (beyond age 60) is another evolving area of study. Earlier studies suggested that age was an important factor in the prognosis for women suffering from ovarian cancer and that older women did not do as well as younger women. This theory has been subjected to more debate as we have recognized an important bias: Older patients generally are not given the same treatment options as those offered to younger patients. In fact, older women tolerate chemotherapy as well as do younger women, and the more important factor to consider is not age but the activity you're able to perform on a daily basis (your **performance status**). It is well recognized that a sicker patient who requires 24-hour home care and cannot walk without assistance will fair worse with chemotherapy than will a healthier patient, regardless of age.

Having said this, it may be wise to tailor therapy for women past the age of 70 and for those in specific situations, such as women with an underlying neuropathy from diabetes or other causes or those having a baseline hearing loss.

Older women tolerate chemotherapy as well as do younger women.

Performance status

a numerical description of how a person is doing in their normal day-to-day life and whether their cancer is impacting on their ability to live normally.

54. Should I be taking any special vitamins?

Your doctor may recommend a multivitamin a day. Anything more than that is generally not necessary. You may want to avoid antioxidants (vitamins that function to inhibit cells from being injured) for reasons already stated. As exists for dietary advice, a lot of information has been circulated regarding vitamin supplementation to help the immune system and even about the use of homeopathic remedies, such as coral calcium and shark cartilage. Unfortunately, there aren't a lot of data to tell whether these homeopathic remedies or vitamin supplements are actually helping you. The major goal is to stay away from things that could eventually hurt you, and you need to discuss and review fully with your doctor all the nontraditional medications before you start taking them.

55. Can I work while receiving treatment?

While the treatment for ovarian cancer is very tolerable, it is generally a good idea to take some time off work when you start treatment, until you know how you will feel while on therapy. There are some patients who will be relatively unaffected by their treatment and will be able to work while on therapy, but others will find that they do not have the energy to devote to both a job and to chemotherapy. Remember that while most treatments are now done as outpatients, they still require a lot of time (carboplatin and paclitaxel, for example, can take 6 hours from start to finish). This is why many women often choose to go on disability while on chemotherapy and concentrate on getting better so that they are more able to return to work in a productive capacity.

It is generally a good idea to take some time off work when you start treatment, until you know how you will feel while on therapy.

Andrea's comment:

The people at the company where I worked were very understanding and supportive, holding my job for me until I was able to return to work. I applied for my state's temporary disability insurance right away, as I knew I would be out of work for at least six weeks after surgery. In the end, I found work too taxing while on chemo and, because my husband's income was enough for us to live on, I did not go back to work. I feel I was fortunate to have this option, because I felt that I needed all my strength to fight. That being said, I know others who welcomed the support and sense of accomplishment that work afforded them and were able to work through treatment. Most important, I think you have to speak frankly to your doctor about your situation to determine when going back to work is right for you.

If you decide not to return to work, talk to your benefit administrator to find out whether you qualify for COBRA, a federal program that enables you to continue on the company's group policy even though you're no longer a full-time employee.

If you think you won't be able to return to work for time for some time, apply for Social Security Disability (SSD) benefits. These benefits are based on the amount you have contributed to Social Security over your working life. The application takes some time to process, so if you think you'll be eligible, apply sooner rather than later so that you can begin receiving benefits as soon as possible. Also, talk to your doctor about your need to apply for SSD, as he or she should be familiar with the paperwork and the need to be your advocate. Get your doctor's support for this and, if you're denied, go through the appeals process, as many are approved this way. Another benefit of getting started with SSD is that after two years on SSD, you will automatically be enrolled in Medicare. Hopefully, however, you'll be well, back to work, and not needing this information.

A word about student loans: If you have outstanding student loans, apply for a temporary disability deferment. That way, the government pays the interest while you're disabled, although your loan is not forgiven. In my case, as I continued being treated past the three years allocated for temporary disability deferment qualification, I had to apply for permanent disability. This was a major psychological hurdle for me, as I did not want to think of myself as permanently disabled. However, the fact of the matter was that I was not able to return to work after three years, so I applied and am currently under review for this option.

In finding a new job after a cancer diagnosis, I have heard of two diametrically opposed positions. Some say to be up-front about your medical history, as checkups may be time-consuming and require you to arrange your work hours creatively. However, you're not required to give your health history and may want your privacy protected. Here, con-sulting a lawyer who specializes in disability and work issues can be a help, as can learning about the Family Medical Leave Act, ERISA, and the Americans with Dis-abilities Act. There is also a Web site devoted to these issues: cancerandcareers.org.

56. Will I still be able to care for my kids while receiving chemotherapy? What about my pets?

You should be able to carry out most normal activities even while on chemotherapy. You should not put aside your goals and needs. In fact, most studies show that some people feel better on treatment than they did when they were diagnosed. You need not sequester yourself from your family or your pets while receiving treatment. You may be more tired, particularly as you near completion of your treatment, and may need some help in taking care of your pets or home respon-sibilities. However, with a little help from your friends and family, you should be able to continue your normal routines. This means, however, that you must *accept* help when it's offered. Many people politely refuse an offer from a friend or family member, thinking they

Most studies show that some people feel better on treatment than they did when they were diag-nosed.

don't want to burden others with their illness, but this habit only makes your difficult task of recovery more difficult that it needs to be. If your family and friends want to help, let them!

57. How will treatment affect my sex life?

A woman's vagina can thin and be prone to irritation considerably due to a lack of estrogen after the ovaries are removed. This can make intercourse uncomfortable due to vaginal dryness. Even more, many women suffer a loss of sexual interest due to the psychological impact of being diagnosed with ovarian cancer, surgical debulking, and the physical manifestations of undergoing chemotherapy, most notably the loss of hair. All of these factors may work together to help dampen any interest in sex. However, this does not have to be the case. With a trusting partner and patience, as one comes to accept her diagnosis and the treatments at hand, it is more common for women to rediscover themselves as sexual persons and, together with a patient and understanding partner, rediscover the power and healing nature of intimacy and ultimately recover a sense of sexuality.

Andrea's comment:

The Vagifem (the low-dose pill you insert into your vagina on a regular basis) has helped a lot, although I did not begin this treatment until after chemo treatment was done. I was very concerned about "vaginal atrophy," whereby the tissues thin out and become very easily chafed. I also found that using a really mild soap (for instance, Dove) to clean myself was not irritating. And then there are such products as "Replens," which help to keep your vagina moisturized, and such lubricants as "AstroGlide" for sexual intercourse. My husband and I continued to have a sex life during my treatment, but there were periods in which, owing to physical and emotional side effects of things (surgery, examinations, chemo, and lack of estrogen), I didn't feel much like having sex.

At one point I did ask for a vaginal dilator, which is basically a set of smaller and larger tube-shaped items to give the vagina ever more strenuous "work-outs." I never even opened the box, although I always meant to. I've had to work at keeping up an active sex life, and my husband has been a help here, being very gentle and patient. I imagined myself using a dildo and vibrator to practice, but I haven't gotten there yet, although it's probably a good idea. Talking to a therapist or sharing your feelings in an all-women group can really help here, too.

The lessening of hormones and the trauma of surgery—and even examinations—sometime made sex seem like the last thing on my mind. However, I found that with practice, communication, a patient husband, some good lubrication, intravaginal estrogen, some sex toys, and some humor, I have been able to resume a relatively active sex life.

I think pampering yourself can go a long way here, too. Treating yourself to a nice long bubble bath, a massage by a professional or just a friend, an evening polishing and buffing, and keeping your skin soft with moisturizers can go a long way to continue feeling soft and feminine. During chemo is an especially important time to love yourself and your body, and taking the time to do these gentle activities for yourself can be rewarding.

58. Is depression common after treatment?

Yes, depression is a common experience for women with ovarian cancer. Once a woman is diagnosed, she may work through a whole gamut of emotions from terror, fear, anxiety, and worry. However, as they begin therapy, a sense of resolve sets in for many women and a determination to do whatever is necessary to beat the cancer soon sets in. Yet as much as a woman looks forward to completing treatment, it is not uncommon for many to feel a sense of depression after treatment has completed. It is often due to a sense of anxiety that nothing is being done once treatment has completed (entering the "watchful waiting" period), and with that, a loss of control over what the future may hold. Many women can work through this with the passage of time, as they become more used to the frequent schedule of follow-up visits. But for some, the end of therapy brings about a sense of sadness and a sometimes overwhelming fear, which can be quite debilitating. If this appears to be occurring, it is very important to discuss such concerns with your physician. After all, no woman diagnosed with ovarian cancer should live the rest of her life paralyzed by fear or depression over what may be.

Andrea's comment:

My husband calls the time immediately after the end of treatment "free-fall." During treatment, I found myself pretty busy and focused on fighting the disease and managing the side effects. I didn't worry too much because the treatments were working and I felt that we were doing the best we could to fight the disease. However, then you're finished—treatment stops, friends and family may forget to treat you like a person in need of special care, and life is

No woman diagnosed with ovarian cancer should live the rest of her life paralyzed by fear or depression.

supposed to get back to normal. But I experienced periods of intense anxiety after treatment was finished, because what did I have now to defend me against recurrence?

One intern, when I was about to enter this after-treatment state, advised me to just forget about the cancer and get back into life. And my surgeon advised us to get out and enjoy life, now that my treatment had worked and I was free from cancer and the treatment. I remember thinking, Yeah, sure, I'll forget it just like that ... but I think the advice was on the right track, although it's taken me a few years to get there. I have since consulted a psychiatrist, who recommended an antidepressant, which has helped me.

I find writing about the experience a little difficult, as I don't even want to remember or think about it all too much—it's still too painful. However, maybe there comes a time when looking back on it, reflecting, and expressing one's feelings about the experience can help. In New York City (and many other cities), there are many cancer groups, including "newly diagnosed" and "posttreatment." The posttreatment time brings its own set of difficulties, because here you are, finished with treatment, starting to rebuild your life without cancer and without chemo to slow you down, but a feeling of insecurity can linger.

Right now, I am coping with this period although, as I look at the calendar, I see I am now almost four months posttreatment. I feel that I should be further on in getting back "out there" than I am. My friends remind me to take care of myself, that I may be fragile for a bit of time, but that my strength will improve with time. I wrote another friend all my list of "should be's" and "should do's" right after treatment, and he wrote me the kindest letter advising me just to "be."

59. When will my hair grow back?

Once you complete treatment with paclitaxel, your hair should start growing back, but certainly you should have noticeable hair growth within three months of stopping treatment. It may take six months, or even longer, to have shoulder-length hair. Do not be surprised or shocked if your hair grows back different in texture, style, or color. It may begin as gray or even white, and in more than a few women, it has come back curly. As you get farther out from treatment, your hair should resume its normal appearance as it was before you started therapy. But patience will be necessary before you get to that point.

Do not be surprised or shocked if your hair grows back different in texture, style, or color.

Andrea's comment:

Losing my hair was pretty traumatic. I had shoulder-length hair before treatment, and it was a difficult day when it first started falling out. My advice is: Cut it short and once it starts falling out, shave your head. Purchase a wig or call Cancer Care for one (see the Appendix); sometimes insurance will partially cover it. I wore my wig very seldom, only when I went to a work-related function, and I was much more comfortable in cotton scarves and soft hats. I wore some eye makeup and lipstick to brighten my face. Find out whether there's a "Look Good, Feel Better" program in your area. This is a workshop where makeup artist volunteers help you to create a good look with makeup and to which cosmetic companies donate products for you to take home and use.

My hair started growing back right after treatment ended, and it was not long before my head was covered with a very short and chic style. Sometimes your hair will come back a little differently, especially at first. Mine was curlier and grayer, but that was just the initial few inches; now it's the same color and texture, as I would have expected without any chemo, and I have a lot less gray than I had immediately after. For a long time, people commented on liking my "postchemo cut," but I've let it grow longer.

60. Will I ever enjoy my own life again?

There is no question that being diagnosed with ovarian cancer will change your life. But this does not mean it must be for the worse. Many women find a renewed sense of spirituality after their diagnosis. In addition, it is not uncommon for a life-threatening diagnosis to shock someone into realizing the important things in life. In this way, being diagnosed with cancer can paradoxically improve your life by reminding you how important you are to you and what an important goal your personal happiness is.

Many women find a renewed sense of spirituality after their diagnosis.

Having said this, it is also common for women to suffer from anxiety over what the future may hold. However, even in this case, time is the best medicine. As you get farther and farther out from treatment, the follow-ups, the blood tests, and the radiology exams become routine and you will be able to find a balance between the "worry" and the "rest of your life" that works best for you.

Andrea's comment:

There are many layers to the cancer experience, and in meditation group we talked about not getting "cancer mind." I would describe cancer mind as forming an attachment to the disease or identifying yourself too closely with it. Yes, I'm sure there is a mind–body connection and, after a cancer diagnosis, nothing is really ever the same. There's a loss of innocence, a loss of any sense of immortality you may have been able to hold onto from childhood. And then there is hair loss, and maybe some weight loss, and possibly fertility and job loss—there's a lot to cope with emotionally.

These losses didn't really begin to hit me for some time after treatment, as I was so focused on fighting the disease and coping with the chemo that I couldn't really process much else. In this sense, too, I think it can hit loved ones even harder, as they are helpless to do anything, although they may be able to take in the psychological impact earlier. When it did finally hit me, I found it difficult but necessary to speak frankly with my partner about my fears. I was trying to protect him but, when I did that, I found that it really created distance between us.

That being said, I also think it's of immense importance to attend a group, because I think you can wear out your friends and family with talking about cancer, whereas in a group you can be really free to speak as much as you need to. The most valuable things I gained from attending groups were a sense of not being alone and meeting two women who became close friends. These friendships are very important to me, because we understand each other so much and can share, listen, and gripe without feeling a need to explain or excuse ourselves.

I think the fear and the frustration that come with your diagnosis and its aftereffects can really inhibit your ability to forget yourself and enjoy life. For me, beginning meditation was the difference between having some psychological freedom and ease and feeling trapped in fear. I cannot emphasize enough the difference it made for me. In it, I was able to find some peace in the midst of the life-threatening struggle. I worked one-to-one with my beloved teacher, the late Gene Fairly, who had coped with a cancer diagnosis himself, in developing a mind-body visualization-based meditation, and I worked within a group.

Writing about the experience has reminded me how crucial this was to my well being, and I am renewing my commitment to meditation. Gene would always say, "If you meditate, you will change." That's true, and you may find more strength of spirit than you were aware you had.

I've learned that I can forget I have cancer when I immerse myself in activities outside my head, which for me is through creative endeavor. I have always made it a goal to keep up with my creative activities during treatment, and that has given me something on which to focus outside the health realm. Sometimes, my entire life in every sense was consumed by the illness. I had to pray a lot, and at turns I asked for peace, strength, courage, forgiveness, and guidance.

In meditation group, we'd talk about people who say, "I just want my life to get back to normal, to what it was before." Meditation practice helped me to see that I not only didn't want to but couldn't go back to what I was before. Personally, I had some areas in my life that needed enlightenment in every sense of the word; although I do still feel anxious and worried at times (and this is a part of my character), I think I know myself better and have a better sense of my own power now. So, in some ways I can enjoy life more. I am not so easily trapped by feeling angry or upset at others, because I have learned that my well-being begins with me and does not depend on other's opinion or treatment of me. This is all, of course, from my personal journey, but you'll find things about yourself that will surprise and encourage you, too.

61. Should I follow a special diet?

There is no special diet routinely recommended for women receiving treatment for ovarian cancer. We often remind women that the cancer is only one part of them, not their entire being. As such, everything in moderation is a good rule of thumb. We typically recommend a heart-healthy diet, low in saturated fats and cholesterol. After all, although one undergoes treatment for ovarian cancer, you must remember that we need to take care of the rest of you too.

Andrea's comment:

I was overwhelmed by dietary advice but, in the beginning, I avoided refined sugar and white flour, trying to eat lots of fruit and vegetables and also animal protein, as I felt I really needed the protein and the iron. I found that eating simply, eating smaller meals and only a few foods at a time, helped me to discover what worked best during treatment. I consulted with a Chinese doctor, too, who advised cutting out the sweets, which has been a challenge for me to keep up. I think there's a case to avoid pesticides and hormone-treated dairy products and meats, as they have an effect on hormones. My opinion is that food is of utmost importance, but none of us is perfect, so learn about nutrition and eat the highest quality food that you can. Food is definitely one important part of a wellness program, so you can look at your time during treatment as a time to learn about nutrition and begin adjusting your habits. Fresh air, clean water, good food, exercise, and some kind of spiritual practice, if you are so inclined, will go a long way to contribute to your health. (Broccoli sprouts are super high in anticancer chemicals, but I've preferred broccoli rabe instead.)

62. How do I manage my emotions?

Perhaps one of the most important messages we can make is to find an outlet for your emotions. It is not good to keep them inside, as those feelings will find some way of coming to the surface. Yes, you must bring your own personal strength to the treatments for cancer, but you don't have to be a superhero. Accept your limitations, cry when you need to, and ask for help when you cannot do it alone. Remember that

Find an outlet for your emotions.

women before you have walked the same road, and as such, consider yourself part of an exclusive club that you never imagined you'd join. But you are a part of a community of women with and survivors of ovarian cancer. If help is needed, all you must do is reach out.

Andrea's comment:

Talk them out, write them out, exercise them out, get them out! Just beginning this writing project made me realize how much I was keeping stored in my head—and in my body, too. Talk to your doctor if your moods are significantly, steadily, and negatively impacting your well-being. There are medications that can ease your way. And again, I cannot stress enough how an active commitment to regular meditation practice can have the extra benefit of regulating and enhancing mood. Share your worst fears and feelings in a group; spend time visiting or being visited by friends. Let people know when you need help or need a laugh. More often than not, people want to be of help to you in the ways that they can.

63. What do I tell my family?

This is an incredibly personal question, but honesty should be the driving principle. Often, the best intentions of trying to protect your loved ones result in feelings of isolation and loneliness on the patient's part, and a sense of helplessness and distance on the part of those of us who love them. Cancer is not a diagnosis that affects only one person; it will affect everyone around you. Instead of trying to handle it alone, take advantage of the support that is likely to be available from family and friends.

The best intentions of trying to protect your loved ones results in feelings of isolation and loneliness.

Andrea's comment:

When I first knew the likelihood of my diagnosis, I called my therapist first and told my husband second. I was so afraid to tell him, afraid of hurting him, causing him pain. Also, I did not tell my family until I was absolutely sure of my diagnosis, which really occurred only after surgery. I didn't want to cause unnecessary worry or pain, especially to my parents. However, looking back, I realize that by asking my sister alone, with my husband, to be there during my first surgery, I put an enormous strain on them. I think in retrospect it would have been better all around to speak plainly and have the burden be shared, for there's strength and comfort in sharing. There were times when I spoke very frankly to my family about it, and they were strong enough to hear me.

Every family situation is different, so I think everyone will have a different way of handling it. However, I think that trying to protect others by keeping them in the dark creates emotional distance. There may be times when you need that, and I find now that I no longer report to friends and family every time I have a scan, because we've learned to let go a bit, to trust that everything will be okay, and if it isn't, we know we can deal with it as we have in the past. I don't know how you would tell children, but I'll tell you that the one person who verbally acknowledged my struggle, during my first summer vacation home after diagnosis and treatment, was my young nephew Andrew Roithmayr, aged 9. He said that he was so happy that I made it, that I and Lance Armstrong were the only people he knew who had survived cancer. I don't think he knew anybody that had had cancer and didn't survive but, given the fear quotient this disease has, it didn't surprise me that he thought of the worst. What did surprise me was the grace and innocence with which he comforted me.

One thing on which my husband and I have come to agree is to "face the facts." I've always preferred getting results from CT (computed tomography) scans directly from the

*doctor rather than reading them myself, unmediated. The
doctor helps to put them in context, and always in the context of a plan. However, when we've been anxious about a
CA-125 result, we just bite the bullet and call and find
out. Not knowing and maintaining a vague feeling of
postponing good or bad news can create more anxiety. So,
my natural tendency to want to put my head in the sand
has been mitigated by my husband's seeing the need to face
things directly. We've learned over the years that although
the situation may seem dire, the overall outcome has been
good. So, we've learned to trust that we will, with the doctors' and God's help, be able to cope.*

64. What insurance and financial concerns must I address after my diagnosis?

It is important for you to review your health insurance
policy to ensure you are covered for surgery, medical
treatment, and, if necessary, second or even third con-
sultations. Navigating the medical system can be both
frustrating and time-consuming, so it is worthwhile to
seek out financial help, which may be available in the
financial services office of your hospital or by speaking
directly to a representative of your insurance policy.
You will need to know what and where you are covered. If you find a doctor that you feel comfortable
with who is not a practicing provider within your
insurance plan, make sure you know what, if any, will
be covered by your primary insurance, and what por-
tion of the bills you are likely to be personally responsible for. Your providers should be able to direct you
toward the right people to speak with when it comes
to billing so you can have some estimate of the charges
you may incur from surgery and, if applicable, from
chemotherapy.

Andrea's comment:

Insurance is one area in which it's important for you, or for someone helping you, to be an advocate. This means being proactive, informed, and organized. Get a copy (either from the insurance company directly or through your workplace) of your insurance policy's "Certificate of Coverage." Read it. Read the fine print. Know your rights and responsibilities (i.e., when you need to get "precertified" for a hospital procedure). Sometimes your doctor's office staff will deal directly with your insurance company regarding preauthorization, so be sure to communicate with your doctor's staff about this. Obtaining precertification (which most often requires only a timely phone call by you or your doctor) is crucial in getting procedures paid for. Without a "precert" number, a claim may be denied even though your insurance company agrees that the procedure is necessary.

Find out whether you have any options to purchase, through your employer, any more comprehensive coverage. If at all possible, don't allow your payments and therefore your coverage to lapse. Once your coverage has lapsed, your insurance company may qualify you with a "preexisting condition," which may not be covered by new insurance. Once you are uninsured, it can be very difficult to get a preexisting condition covered.

Begin immediately by creating files to keep yourself organized. Some suggestions, depending on your type of insurance coverage are:

- Medical bills (different files, such as current and to-be-paid; paid; "in-review"; partially paid; in resubmission; in dispute, appeal, or grievance)
- EOBs (explanation of benefits), statements that you receive from your insurance company outlining the

expenses paid out by the insurance company for services. Make sure you receive the EOBs so that in case a problem arises, you can see how and when payments were made.

- Medical correspondence (different files, for example, correspondence to insurance company, to doctors, letters of medical necessity)
- In-network referrals and precertification numbers
- Out-of-network referrals
- Prescriptions and receipts
- Disability insurance
- Laboratory and test results
- Log of doctors' visits
- List of all doctors with insurance I.D. numbers, phone, fax, address (helpful when requesting referrals)
- Correspondence with your employer (regarding sick leave, etc.)

Keeping paperwork in order and responding to it in a timely and effective manner go a long way toward easing anxiety over the feeling of being overwhelmed that can accompany any serious health issue. Even if you don't have insurance, keeping accurate records can assist you in receiving benefits from governmental and private agencies. You may at times need a lot of patience, fortitude, and perseverance to make the system work for you.

Begin by assuming a good and workable relationship with your insurance company, but be prepared—or have a friend or family member be prepared—to be the "squeaky wheel." Keep a detailed log of any phone calls made to the insurance company and hospital billing department, including the gist of the call, the first and last name of the person with whom you spoke, and the date and time of your call.

Find out whether your plan requires you to stay in network or have the option to go out of network and when you need to get referrals. If your insurance plan requires you to stay in-network, begin by working with your primary-care doctor in receiving the referrals you need. Your primary-care doctor can play an important role as helper and advocate even if he or she isn't directly treating you for cancer. The easiest route here is to stay within the network, and your medical billing matters should proceed smoothly. However, be aware that in some circumstances you may be able to receive out-of-network coverage if you can't find the care you need within network. Ask whether the out-of-network doctor can become part of your plan, whether you can be covered for at least some of the fees, and whether the doctor provides any special expertise or service that would qualify for coverage under your plan. This will entail extra advocacy on your (or your helper's) part and on the part of your medical team.

If your insurance plan won't cover a doctor you'd like to see and if you can afford it, consider investing in a consultation. Once you've determined the best course of treatment, the administration of that treatment (such as administration of chemo, blood tests, CT scans) may be performed routinely, in network.

If you find a procedure or doctor's visit not paid as it should be, resubmit the claim as many times as may be needed. If the bill still isn't paid, ask for a review. (Here, the certificate of coverage and your state insurance department can help you to understand procedures involved in requesting reviews, filing grievances, etc.) Ask your doctor's billing staff to help, and get to know the person handling your bills at your doctor's office.

If you find payment for medicines or procedures denied by the insurance company, find out who exactly is saying no and why. Find out whether your insurance company has assigned you a case worker or medical director, and get their names and contact phone numbers. You have the right to appeal, with the help of your state's insurance commissioner, or to file a grievance if you feel that your case isn't being handled properly. Organizations such as The Patient Advocacy Program, your state's insurance department, and your state's congressmen and senators can help here, too. However, do not allow paperwork to get in the way of your receiving timely care.

If you don't have medical insurance, speak to an oncology social worker from the hospital right away to find out your options. Ask whether you can apply to any state, federal, hospital, or pharmaceutical company programs for financial aid or discount. The federal Hill–Burton Program helps certain hospitals and facilities to provide free or low-cost services. Ask your caseworker whether your facility falls within these guidelines and can offer you assistance. If you're a veteran, you may qualify for special assistance. Also, call the American Cancer Society and Cancer Care for assistance in finding out about financial assistance (i.e., Medicaid, Social Security) for which you may qualify. Above all, have faith that help will be provided, and focus on the immediate need of getting the best health care you can.

If you are denied treatment, contact the American Cancer Society, Cancer Care, and the Patient Advocacy Foundation, and call your state bar association to find out whether any program provides free legal counsel to cancer patients with treatment-denial problems.

Go over medical bills as you receive them, and make sure that you understand them. If need be, go in and speak to someone in the billing department if you have any questions. Sometimes, speaking to someone in person, rather than over the phone, is more effective. If your insurance company is slow in paying your bills and you begin receiving collection notices, try to work together with the hospital billing department and insurance company in resolving such matters. A hospital social worker or case worker can help here, too.

Getting involved in billing and insurance matters can be very taxing and emotional. I learned to limit my time dealing with insurance matters to two hours a day, and I hope that you will not need anywhere near that time. Otherwise—and I've heard this from others—the insurance-billing behemoth can consume you. Be practical and get a little done each day rather than trying to solve all the issues in one go. I also tried to maintain a positive attitude when speaking with the claims department workers and even began ringing a Tibetan bell (ever so softly) at the beginning of each billing conversation to help smooth the way! This worked even better than a tranquilizer for me. Working on these matters can become very stressful and consuming, and it either can serve as a potent and concrete reminder of your health situation or as an unhealthy outlet for anger and frustration. So, keep up your records as best you can, work on problems in a paced and consistent manner, and learn when to stop and not get stressed out.

PART FIVE

Symptom Management

What symptoms occur when ovarian cancer progresses?

What happens if I have severe abdominal pain?

What can I do for fatigue?

More ...

65. What symptoms occur when ovarian cancer progresses?

Ovarian cancer usually grows in the belly, or **peritoneal cavity**. As tumor implants lying on the peritoneum and around the bowels continue to grow, more malignant fluid (ascites) is produced. The combination of cancer growth and ascites will cause the symptoms of bloating; eventually, the volume of tumor inside the abdomen will press on the small and large intestine, causing difficulty with eating. Eventually, these effects may require a hospital admission to administer fluids by vein and bring about temporary relief of the symptoms.

Occasionally, the disease may spread through the blood vessels or lymph nodes and show up in the lungs or liver. If it lands in the lung cavity, the cancer can cause fluid to develop around the lung (pleural effusion), which can cause chest pain and difficulty in breathing. Rarely, patients can present with cancer in their brain, and that can produce changes in personality, decreased ability to think clearly (**cognitive changes**), or seizures.

66. What happens if I have severe abdominal pain?

If you develop severe abdominal pain, it's very important that you immediately consult with your physician or seek care in an emergency room to find a reason for your pain and specifically to rule out an intestinal obstruction. The evaluation will require a physical examination and imaging studies, usually abdominal x-rays and a CT (computed tomography) scan of your abdomen and pelvis. Intestinal obstruction, a very

Peritoneal cavity
the abdominal space.

Cognitive
referring to brain function.

common complication of advanced or recurrent ovarian cancer, may require surgery.

If your physician believes that you might have an obstruction, you will have to go to the hospital. Your doctor may recommend surgery to correct the obstruction. If your pain is severe, you may require morphine or another type of narcotic, which may be offered to you as an infusion pump that allows you to control directly the amount of pain medication you get (**patient-controlled analgesia**).

It's important to realize that abdominal pain does not automatically mean that you have an obstruction. There are other possible causes for pain, and most of them can be managed without having to admit you to the hospital. Some common causes are constipation, kidney stones, or a urinary tract infection. However, an obstruction may become an emergency, and then it requires immediate evaluation to rule it out.

Patient-controlled analgesia (PCA)

a method of providing pain medication through the vein which allows direct control over the amount required to make one comfortable.

67. What can I do for constipation?

Constipation is a very common complaint for women with ovarian cancer. It is typically present at diagnosis and can persist throughout treatments and recurrence. Because ovarian cancer tends to grow along the surface of your bowels, the normal function of the bowel is affected which results in constipation. You may require the use of laxatives and stool softeners, such as senna and Colace. If constipation is related to pain medications or progression of your cancer, these may not work enough. There are other medications your doctor may recommend, including lactulose, magnesium citrate, and enemas, to help with bowel movements.

Andrea's comment:

As constipation can be a side effect of surgery, chemotherapy, pain medication, and antinausea medication, there's a chance you may have to cope with this at some point. My doctors recommended that I begin using a stool softener, such as Colace, with a senna-based product, such as Sennokat, before the predictable onset of constipation. In my case, it would begin a day or two after treatment and continue for two or three days. I used milk of magnesia occasionally if I really needed to. I found this regimen to work pretty well, although I was careful to keep a diary for recording foods and medication so I could look back and see what worked best with my digestive system. Chemo has an effect on all fast-growing cells, including the lining of one's digestive tract, and I found that coping with constipation was an ongoing concern. I think keeping regular is of utmost importance to maintaining a good quality of life.

Drink lots of water, especially during chemo; make sure you keep moving, walking every day if you can; and try to eat foods with fiber, such as fruit, vegetables, and oatmeal. On an on-going basis, after chemo, I struggled with keeping regular and at times took small amounts of aloe, took fiber supplements, drank warm prune juice, and took the medications lactulose and Miralax. Here it's important to keep your tools to a minimum so that you can figure out what works for you, and to speak to your doctor or to a gastroenterologist so you know that the things you are taking are working synergistically.

All that said, I finally found—and maybe it was just time that did the healing—that after almost a year of taking a small dose of Miralax daily, I was able to return to relative regularity through fiber supplementation and an antidepressant. Having a relaxed mind can't hurt!

68. How do I manage my pain?

A primary goal of anyone involved in the treatment of cancer patients is to alleviate pain. It is always important for your doctor to perform a history of the pain, exam, and diagnostic studies to determine the source of your pain. If it is related to your cancer, often it is relieved as the cancer shrinks with chemotherapy. However, the use of narcotics is often essential to help with pain. If your doctor is unsure how to dose your pain medication or if the pain is not being controlled accurately, there are now specialists in pain management that you can see. If the pain is found to be due to a specific site of cancer that is pressing on nerves, your doctor may even recommend radiation to help relieve the pain.

Andrea's comment:

While in the hospital, you should be receiving enough pain medication to be relatively pain-free, especially right after surgery. As time wore on, I chose to try to limit the pain meds because of the side effect of constipation, but who knows whether that small adjustment (I did not go off them entirely) made much of a difference? For me, the worst postsurgical pain was that relating to "gas pains," the cramping that goes along with the return of bowel movements after surgery and anesthesia. I found that lying on the floor, knees bent, and rocking gently side to side while breathing deeply really helped with the gas pains. I did give a scare to the doctor who found me lying on the floor on a blanket, but it got so that the nurse was not surprised to find me there. I think you could do this in the hospital bed too, but it's a little harder to roll on a soft surface.

You should receive enough medication to make your return home relatively pain-free, except for gas pains that can still be uncomfortable by the time you get home. If you're experiencing pain, talk to your doctor and to the doctors in the pain-man-agement department of the hospital. I've read that cancer patients can be undermedicated for pain and that the field of "pain management" is new, so be sure to be vocal about your level of pain and what you need to feel comfortable.

I also found that watching an engrossing drama or comedy and working with my hands (I've learned to knit, crochet, and sculpt in clay) help to alleviate pain by distracting my attentions elsewhere.

69. What can I do for fatigue?

Fatigue is a common side effect of chemotherapy, drug therapy, and of the cancer itself. Many women find their own personal way of coping with it. If you are found to be anemic, often using medications like Epogen (Procrit™) will help by increasing your red cell count, which may help. If you are on chemotherapy, drinking fluids may help by preventing dehydration. Try not to restrict yourself solely to water; use fluids rich in metabolites to replenish important electrolytes that may be lost as your body copes with the chemotherapy. Fatigue may also be a side effect of medications, like the antinausea agents and pain medications. If this is happening to you, talk to your doctor about alternatives that may be available but not cause as much tiredness. Finally, try your best to stay active, even though it may be difficult at first. You may find it becomes easier with time.

Andrea's comment:

Drink lots of water. Keep moving, but don't get overtired. I've found now that after my last course of treatment, I have experienced a degree of "deconditioning," and it's been a little harder to get my strength and stamina back. Again, drink lots of water. Get sleep; use a sleep aid if you need to.

Get some exercise and try to maintain your fitness as best you can without overtiring yourself. I tried to walk or ride my bike everyday during my first course of treatment, and it helped me to maintain muscle mass. On the other hand, as time went on and I experienced a more chronic level of fatigue, I found it a fine balance between resting and building up my "chi" and resting too much and losing strength. At some point, you may hit the wall of fatigue, and there's nothing to do but stop and rest. Learning to pace myself is another lesson I've learned, and I've found that in doing one thing well (even "mindfully"), I enjoy that experience so much more than multitasking or trying to accomplish too much in one day and getting frustrated. Fear and frustration are the enemies of living fully, so do what you can to calm the fear and lessen the frustration.

70. How is ascites treated? What about pleural effusions?

If you have a large-volume ascites when you are first diagnosed, your surgeon will drain the fluid during the primary surgery, removing several liters during the initial operation. This is part of the debulking (resecting or removal) operation that is done at the time of the original diagnosis.

The majority of patients with new ovarian cancer (70–80%) will respond to chemotherapy, and chemotherapy will usually prevent reaccumulation of ascites.

If the cancer does not respond to initial chemotherapy or returns after some time and starts to grow once more, your belly may fill up with ascites again. In that event, doctors use other types of chemotherapy to get control of your cancer, which is the primary way to control the ascites. Often, to control abdominal swelling, your physician may repeatedly drain the ascites using a needle through your abdominal skin (a procedure known as a **paracentesis**). If the swelling is severe, it may cause you to feel full easily when you eat (termed **early satiety**) and uncomfortable when you lie down or may even make breathing difficult.

Paracentesis is not the same thing as surgery. It's usually something that can be carried out at your bedside or with you as an outpatient. Sometimes, if the fluid is in an area that's difficult to reach, your doctor may have to perform the procedure in the radiology department; that way, the radiologist can see where the needle is going into your body and may more accurately drain off the fluid. Unfortunately, although the procedure can relieve you of the symptoms associated with ascites, it's usually temporary; most patients may have to undergo paracentesis once a month or more frequently if the cancer does not respond quickly to chemotherapy.

Fluid buildup around your lungs is called a **pleural effusion**. Sometimes the fluid deposit can become so large that it compresses your lung, which then is unable to work properly. This can cause shortness of breath (**dyspnea**) that is worse when you walk; if it's very severe, it can cause you to be breathless at rest or when you're lying down.

If the fluid starts to interfere with your ability to go about your daily routine without feeling uncomfortable or breathless, your doctor may remove this fluid (a process also called a **thoracentesis**; Figure 4). This procedure is similar to the **paracentesis** discussed earlier. Your doctor would place a needle into your chest cavity and drain the fluid. As will ascites, the fluid likely will return despite being drained. Therefore, to

Paracentesis
the process of removing ascites.

Early satiety
feeling of getting full faster than you normally would.

Dyspnea
shortness of breath.

Thoracentesis
procedure of draining a pleural effusion.

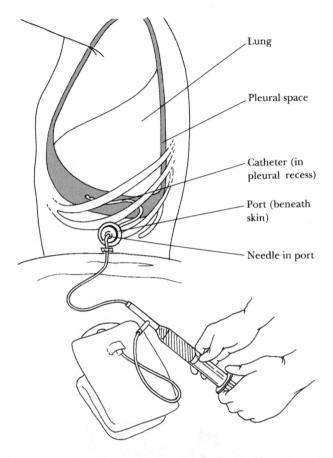

Lung

Pleural space

Catheter (in pleural recess)

Port (beneath skin)

Needle in port

Figure 4   Thoracentesis via an implanted port. Reprinted from Yarbro CH, Frogge MH, Goodman M, Groenwald SL: *Cancer Nursing: Principles and Practice,* **Fifth Ed. Copyright © 2000, Jones and Bartlett Publishers, Inc.**

increase the odds that it will not come back, treating it may require something more permanent.

Once all the fluid is removed, a drug such as talc is placed into the lung space (**pleurodesis**). This agent (drug) prevents further fluid from building up by creating scarring in the space between the chest wall and the lung (which is where the fluid builds up).

Pleurodesis

process performed to prevent further build-up of fluid around the lung.

PART SIX

Relapse

What happens if the cancer comes back?

Can I live with ovarian cancer after it has recurred?

How long will I live?

More . . .

71. How can my ovarian cancer come back if my ovaries have already been removed?

Ovarian cancer cells can escape outside the ovary and be present in many parts of the pelvic and abdominal cavity, particularly in the lining of the peritoneum. They can hide in lymph nodes in any part of your body, or even can show up as microscopic cells in your lung, liver, bone, or brain. Removal of the ovaries will ensure that the original site of cancer is removed, but it does not guarantee that the cancer will not show up elsewhere in your body.

At the time of diagnosis, you may have a small but undetectable volume of cancer cells floating throughout your peritoneum and your entire body; if not treated, these cells may grow and eventually present as a tumor recurrence. This is why most patients with ovarian cancer should receive postsurgical (or **adjuvant**) chemotherapy after surgery. It's a way to secure the destruction of any potential "microscopic metastasis" that may have escaped the ovaries.

72. What happens if the cancer comes back?

If ovarian cancer recurs, your treatment will depend on where the cancer is found and the length of the interval away from chemotherapy (also known as the **treatment-free interval**, or TFI). The TFI is usually measured from the date of the last chemotherapy treatment after your initial surgery to the date of recurrence. In general, if your cancer comes back and requires treatment with another round of chemotherapy within 6 months (after you completed the prior treatment), it's considered unlikely to respond to another round of platinum-based chemotherapy,

Removal of the ovaries will ensure that the original site of cancer is removed, but it does not guarantee that the cancer will not show up elsewhere in your body.

Adjuvant

given after a primary procedure.

Treatment-free interval

time between the end of one chemotherapy regimen to the initiation of a subsequent therapy for recurrent disease.

sometimes referred to as platinum resistance. Your oncologist will generally offer you other chemotherapy drugs that work in a different way, so called **second-line chemotherapy**. Although a repeat surgical procedure may be a possibility, the benefit appears to be in those patients whose TFI is greater than 1 year. Patients whose disease returns after a short time will generally not do as well as those who have a recurrence after a year or more. If ovarian cancer recurs more than 6 months after you complete your chemotherapy, treatment will be based on where the cancer has reappeared and on your TFI.

If the cancer has come back in only one area, surgical removal of the recurrent tumor followed by additional chemotherapy or (in some instances) radiation may be a good option. Alternatively, your oncologist may recommend that you undergo chemotherapy and not surgery, with the goal of having it go into a second remission. Occasionally, recurrent ovarian cancer can be cured with a combination of multimodality treatment that involves surgery, chemotherapy, and even radiation.

73. What do I do if the CA-125 reading starts to rise again?

First, don't panic. Fluctuations of the CA-125 are usual and, because of this, your physician may not be too concerned about a rise, as long as the reading stays within the normal range (in most laboratories below 35). If the CA-125 reading starts to rise but stays in the normal range, it calls for careful observation. This means that your physician may bring you in on a monthly basis as opposed to every 3 months in order to track your marker more closely. If it starts to rise

Second-line chemotherapy
chemotherapy given during recurrence.

Relapse

above normal, it is very important to have the CA-125 repeated and confirmed. If it is confirmed to be going up, you should undergo further evaluation with a CT (computed tomography) scan to see whether the cancer can be seen within your body. Using the CT scan, CA-125, and your physical examination, two scenarios are possible.

The first scenario is that your CA-125 reading is elevated but no cancer is detectable by the CT scan or on physical examination. Often, the CA-125 precedes the cancer's showing up on a CT scan by 2 to 3 months or even longer. The situation in which the CA-125 reading is elevated without any other evidence of cancer is called a **serological relapse**. There is no real standard of how to treat women who have a serological relapse. However, most oncologists agree that chemotherapy in this setting is not called for. They may use other methods to help to slow the rise of the CA-125 or help to delay the cancer from showing up on the CT scan, often by using antiestrogen medications, such as tamoxifen or **letrozole** (see Table 5). In situations such as this, oncologists perform serial CA-125 measurements on a monthly basis and may perform repeat CT scans at more regular intervals (e.g., every 6–8 weeks) to make sure that the cancer is not starting to grow.

Currently, a clinical trial being conducted in Europe is comparing immediate versus delayed chemotherapy for treating serological relapse. The results of this trial will help us to choose the more appropriate recommendation.

The second scenario is that your CA-125 measurement is elevated and the CT scan reveals cancer.

Serological relapse

diagnosis of recurrence solely based on an elevation of a tumor marker without evidence of recurrence by radiology tests.

Letrozole

an anti-estrogen medication.

Table 5   Hormonal agents used in the treatment of ovarian cancer

Estrogen blockers (block estrogen stimulation on tumor cells.
   Tamoxifen

Aromatase inhibitors (block a protein called **aromatase**, which converts adrenal hormones (also known as **androgens**) to estrogens; ultimately leads to estrogen blockade at the tumor cell.
   Anastrazole
   Letrozole
   Exemestane

Gonadotropic-releasing hormone agonists work in the brain on the pituitary gland and causes an initial rise in sex-related hormones—testosterone in men and estradiol in women—but with more frequent administration causes a reduction of circulating hormone levels.
   Leuprolide acetate

Relapse

When the cancer is visible on a CT scan, most oncologists will recommend treatment. The type of treatment will depend on several factors: whether your symptoms are related to the cancer, how much cancer is present, the interval between the end of your treatment and the discovery of the recurrent tumor, and how you're feeling overall. However, in regard to recurrent cancer, you should explore all therapeutic options. They could include the possibility of a second operation to resect (remove) the recurrent cancer, chemotherapy, and perhaps even the use of radiation.

It is important to stress that the CA-125 level is not an absolute measure of how much cancer is in your body. Some women have a large cancer burden but have a low marker reading. Alternatively, some have an elevated CA-125 reading but have either little or no cancer on CT scan or physical examination.

The CA-125 level is not an absolute measure of how much cancer is in your body.

115

The CA-125 measure should be interpreted as a guide that you and your physician can use to monitor the activity of your cancer. The absolute number is not as important as how rapidly it's changing. Studies now show that the rate at which the CA-125 measurement doubles above normal is an important predictor of disease growth.

74. If the cancer comes back, can I still be cured?

Recurrences will happen to many women with ovarian cancer.

Recurrences will happen to many women with ovarian cancer, particularly if they originally were found to have stage III or stage IV disease. However, recurrence does not equal terminal disease. On the contrary, with the many treatment options available to women with ovarian cancer, one can expect to survive the recurrence and experience a second or greater remission or to live with recurrent ovarian cancer as a chronic medical condition.

Rarely, a patient may be found to have recurrence in only one area within the pelvis. In this kind of situation, using a combination of surgery, chemotherapy, and radiation, oncologists can once again treat the disease with the hope of a long remission.

In those patients whose tumor recurs and is found in multiple areas of their abdomen or pelvis (or both) or whose disease has traveled to their lungs, liver, or elsewhere, the cancer is not curable. There is effective treatment that may be able to reduce the volume of disease and even put your disease back into remission. However, a remission does not last for long, and you will likely be in and out of treatment for the rest of your life.

If you're dealing with recurrent cancer, you must refocus your mind from "getting a cure" for the disease to ways of "living" with it. Physicians may make the analogy that ovarian cancer is like diabetes. Although both can be fatal if not treated appropriately, neither should be considered a death sentence, and the potential for living productive lives despite these diagnoses really does exist.

Fortunately, a number of drugs are available to treat ovarian cancer. In fact, physicians can even use some drugs (the **taxanes**, particularly) at different doses and schedules successfully. With appropriate use of these drugs, allowing for treatment holidays when the cancer appears to be under control, patients can expect to live for years.

75. Will I still need surgery?

Surgery for recurrent ovarian cancer is generally reserved for women whose disease recurs more than a year after completing chemotherapy. Usually, it's reserved for patients whose tumors appear to the surgeon to be completely resectable (removable). Often, resectable lesions are single sites of recurrence in the pelvis, abdomen, or even the lungs. The goal of surgery would be to remove the entire volume of cancer, which would provide a better starting point for additional chemotherapy or radiation therapy.

Surgery may also be performed in other settings. For example, if your cancer is causing your bowels not to function well (called a small- or large-**bowel obstruction**), causing you to vomit uncontrollably, surgery may be performed to bypass the area of obstruction. In this scenario, the goal of surgery is not tumor debulking (resection) but to produce relief from the symp-

For example, if your cancer is causing your bowels not to function well (called a small- or large-bowel obstruction).

Bowel obstruction
condition in which the small or large bowel is blocked, due to either adhesions or tumor that cause the bowel to back-up instead of work normally (to get rid of stool).

toms related to the cancer, also known as **palliation**. We discuss more about palliation later.

76. Do hormones have a role in treating the cancer?

Epithelial ovarian cancer is not considered to be estrogen-driven. It's true that estrogen receptors are found on this cancer, but their role in disease spread or recurrence is not as clear. In addition, we know now that the use of estrogen replacement therapy doesn't negatively influence your survival. Surprisingly, though, we also know that hormone blockade can be helpful in the chronic management of ovarian cancer. Such drugs as tamoxifen, which blocks the effects of estrogen on cells, have been used in ovarian cancer patients and in women with advanced disease. Up to 15% of women given tamoxifen will have a response. Oncologists have also used other hormone blockade drugs in the treatment of chronic ovarian cancer (see Table 5).

Nonepithelial ovarian cancers (e.g., granulosa-cell tumors) can also be hormonally driven, and physicians should avoid the use of estrogen. In fact, the drug **leuprolide acetate** (see Table 5) has been shown to be active in the treatment of granulosa-cell tumors.

Leuprolide acetate

an anti-hormone that blocks release of estrogen and progesterone at the level of the brain.

77. Are treatments available if my cancer comes back?

Multiple options are available for treating recurrent ovarian cancer; the choice depends largely on your treatment-free interval (TFI). We know that it's possible to administer platinum-based agents (drugs) with good results in re-treating cancer at the time of its recurrence but that the outcome from retreatment is influenced by the TFI. The response rate can range from 27% if the TFI is 1 year to 77% if the TFI is longer than 2 years.

If you have a TFI of 3 to 6 months, the chance of a response to carboplatin is not that high. In such situations, most oncologists would recommend using a drug that works differently than carboplatin.

Fortunately, many drugs that are active in treating ovarian cancer can be tried. These include liposomal doxorubicin (Doxil); topotecan (Hycamtin); gemcitabine (Gemzar); docetaxel (Taxotere); vinorelbine (Navelbine); hexamethylamine (Hexalen); and etoposide (VePesid; see Table 6). In addition, clinical trials (tests involving patients and experimental drugs) continue to explore new ways of fighting ovarian cancer, and such trials are open to patients throughout the country in cancer centers and major research institutions.

It is important at this point to clarify how drugs are prescribed. There are three types of drugs that might be used to treat ovarian cancer. The first kind is the experimental drugs, which have not been approved for use by the Food and Drug Administration (FDA) and therefore cannot be prescribed outside of a clinical trial, unless a physician gets a "compassionate use" waiver for a patient who has run out of options. The second kind includes all drugs that have completed clinical trials in ovarian cancer patients and were found to be effective; these drugs have been given the stamp of approval for use in ovarian cancer patients, although the approval is sometimes qualified—that is, they may

Table 6   Standard drugs used in chemotherapy for ovarian cancer

Agent	Activity	Route of Infusion	Major Side Effects
Platinum analogs	Cross-link DNA, lead ultimately to DNA damage and cell death		
Cisplatin[A]		By vein every 3 weeks	Nausea, vomiting; numbness, tingling that may not be reversible; kidney injury; hearing loss; ringing in the ears (tinnitus)
Carboplatin[A]		By vein every 3 weeks	Lowered platelet count and white blood cell count; possible infection; nausea (less than with cisplatin); mild numbness, tingling; low risk for hearing problems
Taxanes	Inhibits cells from dividing by binding microtubules		
Paclitaxel[A]		By vein either as 1-hour infusion weekly; 3-hour infusion (if given with carboplatin) every 3 weeks; or 24-hour infusion every 3 weeks (if given with cisplatin)	Allergic reactions; complete hair loss; muscle and joint pain; numbness, tingling (reversed when drug is stopped); lowers white cell count
Docetaxel[O]		By vein as 1-hour infusion, every week or every three weeks.	Allergic reactions; lowered white cell count; hair loss; diarrhea; fluid retention

(continued)

Table 6   Standard drugs used in chemotherapy for ovarian cancer   (continued)

Agent	Activity	Route of Infusion	Major Side Effects
Vinca alkaloids	Stop cells from multiplying by binding cell structures called tubulin		
Vincristine,^{O} vinblastine,^{O} vinorelbine^O		By vein every 2–3 weeks (vincristine, vinblastine); every 1–2 weeks (vinorelbine)	Skin and soft-tissue damage from leaks into skin; numbness, tingling; constipation (severe with vinblastine); nausea; hair loss; lowered white blood cells
Topoisomerase inhibitors	Stabilize DNA with enzyme (topoisomerase), leads to DNA damage and cell death		
Topotecan^A		By vein weekly or daily for 5 days every 3 weeks	Lowered red and white cells, platelets; hair loss, fatigue, or rash (less common)
Irinotecan^O		By vein, usually weekly for 4 weeks, then 2 weeks off (i.e., 6-week cycle)	Significant diarrhea; lowered white cells or platelets hair loss nausea, vomiting lung injury
Etoposide^O		Orally for 3 of 4 weeks	Lowered white cells and platelets; nausea, vomiting; hair loss; leukemia reported in women previously treated with etoposide

(continued)

Relapse

Table 6 Standard drugs used in chemotherapy for ovarian cancer (continued)

Agent	Activity	Route of Infusion	Major Side Effects
Anthracycline antibiotics	Interrupts DNA, leads to cell death		
Doxorubicin[A]		By vein every 3 weeks	Serious tissue injury from intravenous line leak; lowered white cells, platelets; heart failure
Liposomal doxorubicin[A]		By vein every 4 weeks	Painful rash on palms and soles; acute infusion reaction (flushing, chills, back pain, shortness of breath, lowered blood pressure), generally resolves with interruption of infusion
Antimetabolites	Incorporates into DNA and leads to DNA damage and cell death		
Capecitabine[O]		Orally twice daily for 2 of 3 weeks	Lowered red and white cells, platelets; nausea or vomiting; diarrhea or constipation; abdominal pain; rash on hands and feet
Gemcitabine[O]		By vein weekly for 3 of 4 weeks	Lowered white cells, platelets; rash; shortness of breath; flu-like syndrome; mild nausea

(continued)

Table 6   Standard drugs used in chemotherapy for ovarian cancer   (continued)

Agent	Activity	Route of Infusion	Major Side Effects
Antitumor antibiotics			
Bleomycin[O]	Breaks DNA in presence of copper, iron, and cobalt; causes cell death	By vein weekly	Lung toxicity (possibly fatal); fever, oral ulcers; hair loss; skin darkening; anorexia; lowered blood counts
Alkylating agents			
Altretamine[A]	Disrupt DNA, cause cell death	Orally four times daily for 14–21 days	Nausea, vomiting; numbness, tingling; lowered blood cell counts
Melphalan[A]		Orally for 4 days every 4–6 weeks	Lowered blood counts; possible leukemia later in life
Chlorambucil[O]		Orally for 5–14 days	Lowered blood counts; nausea, vomiting; leukemia risk later in life
Cyclophosphamide[A]		By vein every 3 weeks	Nausea, vomiting; lowered blood counts; bladder bleeding (hemorrhagic cystitis); hair loss

[A]FDA approved for use in ovarian cancer.

[O]Approved for other uses but sometimes prescribed off-label for ovarian cancer.

Relapse

be approved for use in one stage of the disease but possibly not for another. The third kind is a gray area: drugs that have been approved for use in a similar disease (for example, breast cancer) but not for ovarian cancer. Such drugs may be prescribed "off-label"—that is, not in accordance with the rather stringent FDA indications—if the physician has reason to believe it might be effective. This is not as much of a "stretch" as it might sound: in many cases, very similar drugs *are* approved for use in ovarian cancer, but the particular drug being prescribed off-label simply hasn't gotten through sufficient trials to ascertain the proper dose, its effectiveness for a given stage of cancer, or that it is more effective and/or less toxic than the standard, approved drugs. Looking at Table 6, you'll see, for example, that the drug paclitaxel is approved for ovarian cancer, while docetaxel is not. Both are taxanes, and both are effective against similar cancers, so it's entirely possible that docetaxel could work against ovarian cancer—but it's not approved. Only by going through (and passing) the rigorous testing required by the FDA will it gain that approval.

It's important to keep in mind that although the goal of treatment for recurrent cancer is to induce a remission of the cancer, and the chance of a permanent remission (cure) for recurrent ovarian cancer does not exist—yet. Do not forget that advances in cancer treatment are occurring continually, so that a new, more effective treatment for recurrent ovarian cancer could be just around the corner. Currently, the aim of treating recurrent ovarian cancer is to prevent or minimize cancer-related symptoms by decreasing the amount of tumor present. The major challenge in choosing a treatment is to choose an active drug that will not cause more symptoms than those caused by the cancer itself.

78. Can I live with ovarian cancer after it has recurred?

Absolutely. Although not curable, recurrent ovarian cancer is treatable. Given the many drugs available, it's possible to find a treatment that will not cause significant side effects and will allow you to live as independently as possible for as long as possible. The survival for women with ovarian cancer continues to improve. Part of living with this cancer is to be realistic about treatment. If you start a new treatment expecting to be cured, you'll often find yourself discouraged and sometimes even depressed. However, if you accept that the cancer will be with you for life, you'll be better able to focus on controlling the cancer and participating in the medical decisions that will affect you and your lifestyle.

Survival for women with ovarian cancer continues to improve.

79. If I can't be cured, why should I undergo chemotherapy for recurrent disease?

Although recurrent disease cannot be cured, it can be controlled. In fact, there's even a chance that your cancer will go back into remission. The natural history of ovarian cancer is one of relapse (recurrence) and remission, often repeating this cycle of relapse and remission, which can translate into survival through the years. Again, recurrent ovarian cancer is not synonymous with terminal disease. Instead, recurrent ovarian cancer can be managed for years as a chronic illness. The use of

Recurrent ovarian cancer can be managed for years as a chronic illness.

chemotherapy allows this, and the judicious use of agents can accomplish it with controllable side effects.

80. Will I be receiving chemotherapy for the rest of my life?

The goal of chemotherapy is to get your cancer back into remission, or at least to keep it from growing. Once your physicians feel that your disease is under control, it's possible for you to have some time between chemotherapy treatments, often called a **treatment holiday**. In general, it's not a good idea to receive chemotherapy on a chronic (constant) basis. Your body can get tired of receiving treatment and this can cause symptoms, such as worsening tiredness; your laboratory studies could reveal such effects as low blood counts that are slow to recover with each successive treatment. Therefore, it's always a good idea to take a break, if possible, to allow your body a chance to recover from treatment.

Another interesting feature of ovarian cancer is that, unlike many other cancers, it can potentially respond once again to the same drugs used previously. This explains why your doctor may recommend treating recurrent cancer with the same drugs (carboplatin and paclitaxel) that you received as adjuvant (or up-front) treatment. However, the most important predictor of our ability to re-treat your recurrent cancer is your treatment-free interval. If you can be monitored off chemotherapy and are able to stay off it for at least 6 months, the chances of another response to carboplatin or to other agents are improved.

Treatment holiday
a break in treatment that allows the body time to recover from toxicity.

81. If my cancer goes into remission, what can I do to increase my chances that it won't come back again?

No standard treatments can maintain a remission. However, the management (treatment) of ovarian cancer in second or greater remission has prompted many different research programs throughout the country to find ways of extending the time of remission. These programs may use chemotherapy or more novel treatments, such as vaccines, to maintain remission.

Andrea's comment:

Try to keep up your healthy habits and exercise to help prevent recurrence and to help to keep you strong in the event of a recurrence. Although we hope this won't occur, if it does, handling surgery, chemo, or other treatments while strong is much easier than to enter a course of treatment in a weakened state. After my last treatment, I have experienced a level of deconditioning that also resulted in some weight gain. So I need to listen to my own advice here and to start to exercise more and eat less—and better.

82. How long will I live now that my cancer has recurred?

This question is the one nearly every patient with cancer asks (or worries about, even if she don't ask it), but it's almost impossible to predict how much time a specific patient will have. The fact is that some women will die quickly from their cancer, while others will live well beyond 5 years, and there's no predicting who will live longer and who won't. Some patients given prognoses of a few months live for years longer than their

It's almost impossible to predict how much time a specific patient will have.

Relapse

doctors expected. Most clinical trials show that survival from a diagnosis of recurrence ranges from 40 to 84% at 3 years. However, we must emphasize that many factors must be taken into consideration for each individual patient. You shouldn't try to apply these statistics to your specific cancer and situation. Remember, too, that your doctor's prognosis of "two to three years" is made without any knowledge of future scientific breakthroughs. There are plenty of people alive today whose doctors predicted short lifespans for them initially—people whose lives were saved by the creation of new forms of cancer therapy that work well on even advanced cancers. So take any predictions about your future with a big grain of salt, because medicine, like everything else, changes very rapidly.

Dealing with recurrent cancer is about more than simply living as long as possible, however. An important aspect of the prognosis is knowing how much *good* time you have left to you, also referred to as "quality of life." We can improve and lengthen your "good-quality life" by offering chemotherapy to control your cancer from spreading and to limit cancer-related symptoms; by making sure that any pain you have is addressed fully; by using every means necessary to ensure that your bowels continue to function; and by knowing when further therapy is likely to hurt you more than help you. All this must be done in the setting of an open and honest relationship.

PART SEVEN

If Treatment Fails

Does intravenous feeding play a role?

What is hospice?

What are the end stages of ovarian cancer like?

More . . .

83. How do I know when it's time to stop treatment?

The relationship between you and your oncologist is very important and must be built on honesty and trust. This becomes more and more important if you're dealing with recurrent ovarian cancer, particularly as different treatments become necessary to try to control your cancer. Because this is a cancer that can be controlled in many women, most patients will undergo several regimens of chemotherapy with the hope of sending the cancer into remission or at least stopping it from actively growing. In fact, it's not uncommon for patients to receive three or even more different types of chemotherapy during the course of their cancer.

One of the hardest questions to ask—and even harder to answer—is when to stop trying.

One of the hardest questions to ask—and even harder to answer—is when to stop trying. Sometimes, a patient will become too sick for further treatment, in which case the oncologist would recommend stopping. Other times, it's the patient who refuses further treatment and instead chooses to live out the rest of her life naturally.

For the majority of patients, the time to stop may be on realizing that, after multiple rounds with different types of chemotherapy, the cancer has only continued to grow and no promising agents are being used in a clinical trial (a test involving patients and drugs). However, ultimately you and your physician must make the decision to stop. If patients in this type of situation still maintain an independent lifestyle, continuing other types of novel treatment or chemotherapy may be reasonable.

If a patient's bowels stop working, particularly if this happens after or during one of these drug regimens (programs or schedules), doctors should discontinue treatment. The reason is that chemotherapy cannot relieve a bowel obstruction, but it certainly can add to its complications.

84. What is a PEG tube? Do I need one?

A PEG tube is a **percutaneous endoscopic gastrostomy** tube. The name describes how and where it's placed. A stomach specialist or **gastroenterologist** would place it during a short procedure. Usually, your doctor would give you medication to make the insertion more comfortable, but it does not require that you be put to sleep, as with regular surgery.

During the procedure, the gastroenterologist will use a special fiberoptic camera, called an **endoscopic camera**, introduced through your mouth and into your stomach. Once it's in place, the specialist would pump air into your stomach so that when a light shines in the internal stomach, it can be seen outside, through the skin overlying it. The specialist would make a hole through the skin and into your stomach and, through this hole, would place a tube by passing it over the camera. It remains in place in your stomach and exits through the hole in your skin.

The main purpose of a PEG is to provide continuous stomach drainage in patients who have a bowel obstruction due to cancer growing around the small intestines and in whom surgery cannot be performed for technical reasons. A PEG is not placed in everyone who has ovarian cancer. It's usually reserved for patients whose cancer is very advanced and who suffer from continual vomiting caused by gastric juices backing up from the bowels because of an intestinal

Percutaneous endoscopic-gastrostomy (PEG)
a tube placed by a gastroenterologist that is inserted through your skin (percutaneous) and into your stomach using a flexible tube containing a camera (endoscopic). A hole is made in the stomach (gastrotomy) and the tube is fixed from the stomach and exits the skin. The purpose is to allow continuous drainage of bowel contents in a woman with terminal cancer who has an intractable bowel obstruction.

Gastroenterologist
a medical specialist in treating disorders of the esophagus, stomach, bowel, and rectum.

Endoscopic camera
a flexible camera within a tube (the endoscope) that is used to do minimally invasive procedures.

obstruction (blockage). The PEG allows the fluid to exit the body more easily, which helps the patient to stop vomiting.

The PEG tube is usually permanent and is attached to a drainage bag into which the stomach contents are drained continuously. Women who have PEG tubes can continue to drink liquids; but whatever is not absorbed into your bowel exits through the PEG tube, instead of coming back up as vomit. Women with PEG tubes can also enjoy independence, since the bag to which the PEG tube is attached can be attached to the patient's leg.

The PEG tube is not a treatment for cancer; it's a way to relieve vomiting due to malignant intestinal obstruction, so that you're not throwing up all the time. Sometimes, if you're feeling better, your doctor might disconnect the tube so that you can take pills and eat and drink. However, if you were suddenly to feel nauseous, the tube can be allowed to drain so that you're not throwing up.

It's important to realize that not all patients require a PEG tube. It's offered only as a way to live with the cancer when it's far advanced and the treatments are no longer keeping it under control. As a consequence, it's used only in the most advanced cases when the disease is considered terminal.

85. Does intravenous feeding play a role?

Total parenteral nutrition (TPN)

nutrition that is given by vein.

Intravenous feeding, or **total parenteral nutrition** (TPN), is usually reserved for women when they first get sick with their cancer. Surgeons use TPN to help to provide nourishment to their patient to make the aggressive up-front treatments of surgery and chemotherapy more manageable.

However, the role of TPN for women with recurrent ovarian cancer is more controversial. If the cancer is growing to the point at which the patient can no longer eat or drink, TPN is probably of very little value. Its use requires an indwelling (permanently placed) intravenous line or mediport and can cause complications (e.g., clotting) due to the catheter, metabolic problems, and infections. More important, it has not been found to improve the life span of advanced cancer patients, nor has it been shown to offer much in the way of relieving hunger or thirst. In one study of patients with different types of cancer receiving TPN, patients with ovarian cancer given home TPN had the shortest survival, compared to similar patients with colon cancer or appendiceal primaries.

In individual situations, TPN may be offered, but that option must take place only after a thoughtful discussion among you, your family, and your doctor. Such a frank discussion should take into account the pros and cons of TPN in the context of how you're doing at the time.

86. What is hospice?

Hospice is otherwise termed **palliative care** or end-of-life care. When treatments are no longer working and a patient becomes very sick because of her cancer, the doctor may recommend hospice. It represents a concerted effort by doctors and other health care providers to recognize that the end of life is a part of the disease process. We have a responsibility to help the patient and her family to remain as comfortable as possible, with dignity and free of pain. Hospice care can be delivered either in an inpatient facility (either a hospital or nursing home–type setting) or at home.

Palliative care
care to provide relief of pain.

Often, providers make an attempt to honor the wishes of a patient. If a woman chooses to go home to live out the rest of her life, providers can set up hospice services to meet her needs and address issues of pain and comfort. They also try to take into the account the concerns of the family. However, if the patient's needs are too much for the family to handle or if she's too sick to go home, her health care providers may recommend inpatient hospice. The ultimate goal is to provide a peaceful death when a patient reaches the end stages of cancer.

87. What is a DNR order?

DNR stands for "Do Not Resuscitate." This order represents your wishes in case something happens to you that without the use of machines, you would likely die. If you were unable to speak for yourself, these wishes will help your family, your physician, or your health care proxy to make decisions for you when that time comes. In this order, you would be asked to state specifically what you would want done and what you would not want done if you were to have a life-threatening event.

These decisions are in large part state-determined. For example, in Connecticut, a DNR order must specify clearly if you do or do not want to have a tube inserted into your throat to help you breathe (**intubation**), cardiac resuscitation, intravenous fluids, or total parenteral nutrition (TPN). In New York, both intubation and cardiac resuscitation are included in the DNR order.

Intubation

process by which a person is placed on a breathing machine.

The best time to discuss a DNR order is when you are still healthy. A DNR order is not permanent.

You should not wait to establish a DNR order until you become so sick that you have to make the decision without having time to really think about it or you are considered terminal. The best time to discuss it is when you are still healthy, so that you and your family can ask questions and thoroughly talk it over with your doctor.

It's important to realize that a DNR order is not permanent. If at any point you change your mind regarding what you would want for yourself in a life-threatening situation, your health care team and your family must respect your wishes.

88. What is a health care proxy?

A health care proxy is a person whom you designate to make health care decisions for you in the event that you are unable to tell your physicians your wishes. This can be a very important role, so it's important for you as a patient to initiate a discussion of what you would want for yourself. Only then can your physicians make sure that they're abiding by your wishes. If you don't designate a health care proxy, your family often has to make decisions for you. Doing that can be risky because, although they may be acting with your best interests at heart, their decisions may not necessarily be what you would want. In addition, it's not uncommon for different members of your family to disagree with each other, particularly when it comes to someone they love. By designating a health care proxy, your family and loved ones would know that you specifically chose someone to speak for you.

89. What are the end stages of ovarian cancer like?

Ovarian cancer usually causes problems by spreading throughout the abdomen and pelvis. Although cancer can involve the brain, lungs, and liver, most women die of disease affecting their bowels. Obstruction of the large bowel (the **colon**) can lead to problems with bowel movements, causing constipation. This can cause the colon to become very large, much like a balloon, also called **colonic dilation**. If it persists, it can become an emergency and result in a tear in the bowel, called a

If Treatment Fails

By designating a health care proxy, your family and loved ones would know that you specifically chose someone to speak for you.

Colon

the large intestine, part of your gastrointestinal tract. The function is to absorb water and food and to excrete stool.

Colonic dilation

the end process of a bowel obstruction where the bowel essentially bursts because neither food or gas can move.

Perforation

bowel injury in which a hole is caused, usually as a result of bowel obstruction, surgery, or infection.

Nasogastric (NG) tube

a tube placed temporarily through the nose (naso) into the stomach (gastric) to help relieve continuous vomiting caused by a bowel obstruction.

Ureters

the anatomical structure that enables us to get rid of urine. It connects the kidney to the bladder.

Hydronephrosis

abnormal enlargement of the kidney.

Hydroureteronephrosis

abnormal enlargement of the kidney and the tube where urine flows, called the ureter.

Fistulas

abnormally formed channels between two otherwise separate organs, such as between the vagina and bladder (vesicovaginal) or between the bowel and the skin (enterocutaneous).

perforation. In that event, a surgeon may recommend emergency surgery to deal with the obstruction.

The cancer can also obstruct the small bowel and result in problems when the patient tries to eat. This results in nausea and vomiting of food; if not eating, a patient may also vomit up bile. This, too, can be very painful and may require a **nasogastric tube** (see Question 78) initially and a PEG tube (discussed in detail in Question 84) if it does not resolve.

Tumor growth in the belly can also block the flow of urine. When the urine backs up into the kidneys, the kidneys and the tubes that attach the kidneys to the bladder (the **ureters**) can become enlarged, called **hydronephrosis** if only the kidneys are enlarged or **hydroureteronephrosis** if the ureter is also involved. Although this condition can cause some pain, it may not cause any symptoms at all. However, it can cause the kidneys to stop working if it goes on for a long time. Other problems can include the development of channels between the bowel and the skin or bladder, called **fistulas**.

PART EIGHT

Prevention, Screening, and Advocacy

Can I protect myself from getting ovarian cancer?

Can ovarian cancer be inherited?

Is there any way to screen for ovarian cancer?

More ...

PREVENTION

90. Can I protect myself from getting ovarian cancer?

The only way to prevent against developing ovarian cancer is to have your ovaries removed. However, for women who want to have children or at least want the option to have children in the future, that's not an option. Also, because this is a relatively uncommon disease, there's a strong possibility that a lot of women who would never have gotten ovarian cancer would go through the procedure unnecessarily. Right now, having your ovaries removed to prevent ovarian cancer (termed a **prophylactic oophorectomy**) is reserved for women considered to be at high risk for developing ovarian cancer. Oral contraceptives, or birth control pills, can provide protection against the development of ovarian cancer.

Prophylactic oophorectomy

removal of a woman's eggs in an attempt to reduce or remove a risk for cancer in the future.

91. Can I get ovarian cancer if I've had my ovaries removed?

Technically speaking, having your ovaries removed will prevent you from getting ovarian cancer. However, removing your ovaries cannot prevent **primary peritoneal cancer**, which behaves similarly and is treated in the same way. It turns out that the cells that line the peritoneum are the same cells that line the ovaries. Thus, cancer can arise out of the peritoneal lining. Although this cancer is much rarer than ovarian cancer, having your ovaries removed can't prevent it.

Primary peritoneal cancer

cancer that arises from the lining of the gut, or the peritoneum. This cancer behaves similarly to ovarian cancer, and is treated much in the same way.

92. Will fertility drugs increase my risk of ovarian cancer?

Although taking fertility medications is suspected of increasing one's risk of ovarian cancer by causing your ovaries to make more eggs, no conclusive evidence suggests that this is true. Certainly, there is a concern that hyperstimulation of the ovary can predispose to the development of ovarian cancer, owing to the frequent shedding of the ovarian surface, but this has yet to be proven.

SCREENING

93. Can ovarian cancer be inherited?

Yes, ovarian cancer can be inherited, but it's important to know that the majority of cases of ovarian cancer are not inherited. In fact, estimates figure that only 10% of all ovarian cancers are hereditary.

Generally, a hereditary cancer syndrome is suspected if, at the age of diagnosis, a patient is younger than age 40; has a history of prior breast cancer; or has a strong family history of other cancers, particularly in the immediate family. This having been said, certain well-recognized cancer syndromes run in families and are associated with an increased risk of ovarian cancer.

The most common hereditary cancer syndrome is the hereditary breast-ovarian cancer (HBOC) syndrome. If three or more cases of cancer are found within your immediate family (**first-degree relatives**) along with a history of four or more early-age breast cancer or a history of ovarian cancer at any age, clinically your family has an HBOC syndrome. Most of the cases of this syndrome are due to mutations in one of two

First-degree relatives

blood relatives of your immediate family (father, mother, sister, or brother).

genes, called BRCA-1 and BRCA-2. The BRCA-1 gene has been found on chromosome 7; BRCA-2 is located on chromosome 13. The mutations within these genes may confer a risk for different types of cancers, but both are specifically associated with an increase in breast and ovary cancer.

In addition to breast and ovarian cancer, these mutations are associated with an increased risk of other cancers. BRCA-1 mutation carriers may have an increased risk of colon cancer and prostate cancer (in men). BRCA-2 mutation carriers have an increased risk of male breast cancer, prostate cancer, malignant melanoma, and cancers of the pancreas, colon, gallbladder, and stomach.

Another syndrome found to exist in certain families is termed the Lynch II syndrome, which is a subtype of hereditary nonpolyposis colon cancer (HNPCC) syndrome. Such families contain multiple family members with colon cancer and cancers of the uterus. However, in addition to harboring these two, they are known to have members who have had breast cancer, ovary cancer, and other types. These include cancers of the brain, stomach, and small bowel; leukemias; and sarcomas. The HNPCC syndrome is associated with mutations in human mismatch repair genes that are responsible for correcting errors or mutations in our DNA.

The final type of cancer syndrome associated with ovarian cancer is termed a **site-specific ovarian cancer syndrome**. This syndrome is seen in families with multiple members who develop only ovarian cancer. Researchers have not completely worked out the genetic explanation for this syndrome, although a proportion of these tumors may end up being due to

BRCA-related mutations. Although these families' members have only ovarian cancer, their female members are still considered at risk of breast cancer.

94. Should I have genetic counseling? How do you determine who should go for genetic testing?

If you have a family history of ovarian or breast cancer (or both) or a personal history of breast cancer diagnosed at a young age, you're at increased risk of ovarian cancer. For you, genetic counseling makes sense, especially if you have sisters or young children and you're worried they may have inherited a gene mutation. In addition, if you have a strong family history of multiple types of cancers, getting genetic counseling may make sense.

If you have two first-degree (immediate family) relatives (i.e., mother and sister) affected with ovarian or breast cancer, your probability of having a genetic mutation increases dramatically. The same is true if you or a first-degree relative have had both breast and ovarian cancer. A family history of colon cancer or colon polyps and ovarian cancer also raises your possibility of having a gene mutation. Finally, if your extended family history includes multiple affected members with varying types of cancer, including ovarian cancer, you may want to obtain genetic testing. If you are still unsure, it's always worthwhile to discuss genetic counseling with your doctor.

If you have a strong family history of multiple types of cancers, getting genetic counseling may make sense.

Unfortunately, being told that you have a genetic mutation associated with a cancer risk is often a double-edged sword. It may raise issues within yourself or your family as to what can be done about this risk. Should you have your breasts removed to prevent breast cancer? If you don't have ovarian cancer, should you have your ovaries removed? These surgeries when done to prevent cancer are termed **prophylactic** procedures. Working through such issues is difficult and makes a genetic counselor all the more important so that you can fully understand the risk of cancer in your specific situation and the potential pros and cons of prophylactic surgery.

Notably, recently published reports suggest that prophylactically removing the ovaries in women who have BRCA mutations may decrease the risk of future breast or ovarian cancer.

95. Is there any way to screen for ovarian cancer?

The quick answer to this question is that there are no *worthwhile* screening tests for ovarian cancer for the general population. The worth of a screening program depends on three factors: the sensitivity of the test, which is the probability that a test result will be positive in a person with the disease, called the **true positive rate**; the specificity of the test, or the probability of a negative test result in a patient without the disease, called the **true negative rate**; and the prevalence of the disease, or the number of cases seen in a year. These three factors will determine the predictive value of the test.

True positive rate

the proportion of patients who have a positive test results and who do have the disease.

True negative rate

the proportion of patients who have a negative test result and who do not have the disease.

Some physicians use annual CA-125 tests and transvaginal ultrasound to look for signs of cancer in women known to be at risk. However, neither of these tests is based on good evidence, only on expert opinion. Although its accuracy has been established, the sensitivity of transvaginal ultrasound has to be taken in the context of the incidence of ovarian cancer, which is low in the general population. Thus, the predictive value of a positive ultrasound is less than 10% and increases to only 27% if combined with an elevated CA-125 result. Furthermore, screening for ovarian cancer has not been shown to result in a decrease in the mortality rate from the disease, and there remains a high risk of false-positive results.

Thus, researchers have not recommended screening in the general population. Current research is focusing on the value of screening in a group of women considered to be at high risk for ovarian cancer and on other mechanisms of early detection, including the use of novel serum markers or the use of proteomic profiling. All that being said, for a woman at high risk, serial CA-125 and ultrasound every six months are commonly performed, but the benefit of this strategy still remains to be seen.

96. What kind of research is being carried on to cure this cancer?

The research being conducted in this field is extensive. Major efforts are under way to improve the early detection of this cancer so that we may pick it up when it hasn't spread and hence can more likely be cured. Some of this work is exploring novel markers that may one day replace the CA-125 test as a more reliable and earlier indicator of ovarian cancer. Others are exploring the newer technologies of gene profiling (**genomics**) and protein profiling (**proteomics**) that may tip off doctors to the presence of cancer, even before it can show up on imaging tests.

Genomics
the study of gene expression patterns.

Proteomics
the study of protein profiles.

Work is also being done to improve surgery for ovarian cancer. Gynecological oncologists are leaders in laparoscopic surgery that may one day be an option for surgical staging (discussed in Question 15). Others are looking into more aggressive surgical operations that could obtain a higher number of women whose tumors can be optimally resected.

In addition, we continue to look for better ways to monitor our patients. The work on better imaging techniques, such as the role of PET scans, will help us in that process, particularly when the CA-125 test is not a marker of some patients' cancer. Also, the search for more effective cancer therapies continues. One day we hope to be able to use a pill that will specifically target the cancer and not the surrounding tissue; our hope is to make the delivery (administration) of chemotherapy more convenient and, more important, to reduce its side effects and toxicity. Further, work continues on defining other approaches to fighting cancer, such as drugs that target new blood vessels that may feed a tumor (so-called **antiangiogenesis** agents), drugs that target the proteins that may cause the cancer to resist treatment, and newer drugs that may one day enable us to cure ovarian cancer.

Finally, researchers continue to explore ways to enable the immune system to recognize the cancer cell as foreign, so that it can kill cancer by itself. Investigators recently showed that the presence of immune cells (**T-cells**) in the cancer points to a better prognosis for patients than that obtained from tumors without T-cells. This finding supports the hypothesis that the immune system plays a role in trying to defeat or con-

Antiangiogenesis
to block new blood vessel formation.

T-cells
cells involved in our immune system.

tain cancer and points to another mode of treatment that can be explored.

97. Should I research and learn more about the disease and its treatment?

When you are diagnosed with ovarian cancer, you may find yourself becoming an advocate by default—your own advocate! Indeed, it is our hope that you are reading this book because you want to know *how* to be proactive in your own care. When it comes to ovarian cancer it is useful to know what you are faced with, and that is part of why this book was written. But it also helps for you to be aggressive about gathering information and asking questions. So our immediate answer to this question would be, yes, you should learn more... but do so at your own pace. Don't feel you need to become an expert overnight. Remember, too, that your emotions about your diagnosis should not be shunted aside as you pursue your ovarian cancer education. Take it slowly enough that you can absorb the information and grow comfortable with it before you continue.

As you grow more knowledgeable and become closely involved in your treatment, you may also find yourself becoming an advocate for others. Perhaps you will join a support group and offer support, advice, or just a badly needed ear for someone who needs to talk. Just as teachers learn their subject better through teaching, this sort of advocacy can help you as well as help others. If you want to take it a step further, consider volunteering for an advocacy organization such as those listed in the Appendix, where you can work to raise awareness of the disease or lobby for funding in support of research. If you have the energy and the inclination for this activity, it can prove helpful not only to ovarian cancer patients in general, but also to you specifically. For instance, you would be in a position to know of advances in treatment when they first become available, rather than waiting for your doctor to hear of them and recommend them to you. Again, this depends on how you as an individual feel about these activities; public advocacy is not for everyone, no matter what its advantages.

Whatever road you take, be it personal education or public advocacy, be aware of one drawback: There is so much information and so much data out there that it is not uncommon for women to get lost in the statistics. It is all too easy to forget that statistics are generalizations about ovarian cancer that, like most statistics, are so broad that they are meaningless for an individual. Take them too seriously, and you may find them overwhelming. As Andrea mentions below, educating yourself can be a difficult task. Try to find methods that will work for you without making you anxious or depressed about your disease.

Andrea's comment:

I was lucky in that I have a friend, Marjan Moghaddam, who is an über-master of medical Web research, and she helped us in printing out relevant articles that helped us to be informed. She also gave me the encouragement to seek the best possible treatment, to ignore "statistics," and to cultivate a positive attitude. Being somewhat detached, she was able to face the situation more squarely than I was. Her support, encouragement, and skill were invaluable during the difficult first few weeks.

I found that I didn't enjoy researching the disease and, because I had access to so many support groups in New York City, that I didn't depend on on-line resources such as the ones we mention in the Appendix. I imagine that these could be invaluable to someone who lived in a more remote area. I skimmed what my friend researched for me, and we always had plenty of questions for the doctor. I think it helped us to feel that we had some power over the situation and that we were an active part of the medical team.

I think too that some people are more natural researchers and advocates, and that all patients can strive to take responsibility for making their health care decisions to the best of their ability. And I am convinced that more knowledge and awareness, among women and doctors, would result in many earlier diagnoses of ovarian cancer.

98. Where can I get support?

You can consider a cancer diagnosis sort of like an invitation to join an exclusive women's club that you never expected or desired to join. This is an important concept because it relays a very important message: YOU ARE NOT ALONE. An entire community of women live with and fight this cancer; they are in a situation similar to yours, no matter where you are along the cancer path; and they are available to you for advice, support, or just helping with the day-to-day struggles of life with cancer. In addition, support groups are available in most local communities—for you, your family, and your friends—because we who treat cancer know that this is a disease that not only has an impact on a patient but on everyone who cares about her and loves her. Your nurses are often the best source of information, and they should be able to direct you toward these support groups locally or to a

Your nurses are often the best source of information.

therapist, in case you need to talk things out in a safe and private environment. As cancer care providers, we're here not only to help you manage your cancer but to help you deal with the fear and questions that accompany it.

99. When should I ask for help?

Being diagnosed with ovarian cancer is an incredibly scary process, and no one should go through it alone. If you're feeling isolated and scared, you should reach out for support. Sadness and anxiety are common in women who have just been told that they have cancer. Most women tell me that they feel it's a death sentence and only remember what they read about Gilda Radner's brave but short struggle with this cancer. If you don't discuss them, the fears can build and make the work that must be done too hard. They can also cause a worsening sense that you're alone, and that feeds into a cycle of deepening despair. If this describes what you or someone you love is going through, reach out for help.

Such feelings must be brought out into the open. Anyone diagnosed with ovarian cancer must *want* to fight it and must trust that treatments are available and successful and can give you back your life. Even if the cancer comes back, there's reason to be hopeful.

Often, antidepressant and antianxiety medications are necessary to help you to come to grips with a cancer diagnosis and the change it requires in your life. Medications to help you handle the diagnosis, its challenges, and treatment are not signs of weakness. There are resources available to enable you to regain control of your life so that you can handle the decisions important to fighting this disease.

100. Where can I get more information?

Many resources are available for women newly diagnosed or living with a diagnosis of ovarian cancer. These include the organizations, web sites, and books listed on the following pages. Many more resources are available besides those listed here; check your local library or Amazon.com for books, or go to any of the following organizations' web sites and search for links or resources related to ovarian cancer.

Organizations

American Academy of Medical Acupuncture
4929 Wilshire Boulevard, Suite 428
Los Angeles, CA 90010
Phone: 323–937–5514
Web site: www.medicalacupuncture.org

American Cancer Society
1599 Clifton Road
Atlanta, GA 30329
Phone: 800–ACS–2345
Web site: www.cancer.org

American Society of Clinical Oncology
1900 Duke Street, Suite 200
Alexandria, VA 22314
Phone: 703–299–0150
Web site: www.asco.org

Cancer Care, Inc.
275 Seventh Avenue
New York, NY 10001
Phone: 212–712–8400 (Admin); 212–712–8080 (Services)
Web site: www.cancercare.org.
Page specific to ovarian cancer: www.cancercare.org/types/ovarian/index.asp

Cancer Research Institute
681 Fifth Avenue
New York, NY 10022
Phone: 800–99–CANCER (800–992–2623)
Web site: www.cancerresearch.org

Centers for Disease Control and Prevention
1600 Clifton Road
Atlanta, GA 30333
Phone: 404–639–3534
Toll-free: 800–311–3435
Web site: www.cdc.gov

Department of Veterans Affairs
Veterans Health Association
810 Vermont Avenue NW
Washington, DC 20420
Web site: www.va.gov
Phone: 202–273–5400 (Washington, DC office)
Toll-free: 800–827–1000 (Local VA office)

Fertile Hope
P.O. Box 624
New York, NY 10014
Web site: www. fertilehope.org

Gilda's Club Worldwide
322 Eighth Avenue, Suite 1402
New York, NY 10001
Phone: 888–GILDA–4–U
Web site: www.gildasclub.org

Gynecologic Cancer Foundation
401 N. Michigan Avenue
Chicago, IL 60611
Phone: 312–644–6610
Fax: 312–527–6658
Web site: www.wcn.org/gcf

Health Insurance Association of America
555 Thirteenth Street NW, Suite 600
East Washington, DC 20004–1109
Web site: www.hiaa.org
Phone: 202–824–1600

Appendix

Health Resources and Services Administration–
Hill-Burton Program
Health Resources and Services Administration
U.S. Department of Health and Human Services
Parklawn Building
5600 Fishers Lane
Rockville, MD 20857
Phone: 301–443–5656
Toll-free: 800–638–0742/1–800–492–0359 (From the Maryland
  area)
Web site: www.hrsa.gov/osp/dfcr/about/aboutdiv.htm

Institute of Certified Financial Planners
Phone: 303–759–4900
Toll-free: 800–282–7526 (Automated referral service)
Web site: www.icfp.org

National Cancer Institute
National Cancer Institute Public Information Office
Building 31, Room 10A31
31 Center Drive, MSC 2580
Bethesda, MD 20892–2580
Phone: 301–435–3848 (Public Information Office line).
Web site: www.nci.nih.gov
National Cancer Institute's Cancer Trials site lists current clinical
  trials that have been reviewed by NCI:
  http://cancertrials.nci.nih.gov

National Center for Complementary and Alternative Medicine
NCCAM Clearinghouse
PO Box 7923
Gaithersburg, MD 20898
Phone: 888–644–6226
Web site: www.nccam.nih.gov

National Comprehensive Cancer Network
50 Huntingdon Pike, Suite 200
Rockledge, PA 19046
Phone: 888–909–NCCN (888–909–6226)
Web site: www.nccn.org

National Ovarian Cancer Coalition, Inc.
500 NE Spanish River Boulevard, Suite 14
Boca Raton, FL 33431
Phone: 561–393–0005
Toll-free: 888–OVARIAN
Fax: 561–393–7275
Web site: www.ovarian/org

National Viatical Association of America
1200 Nineteenth Street, NW
Washington, DC 20036–2412
Phone: 202–429–5129
Toll-free: 800–741–9465
Web site: www.nationalviatical.org

National Women's Health Information Center
8550 Arlington Boulevard, Suite 300
Fairfax, VA 22031
Phone: 800-994-9662
Web site: www.4women.gov

Office of Minority Health
P.O. Box 37337
Washington, DC 20013-7337
Phone: 800-444-6472
Web site: www.omhrc.gov

Ovarian Cancer National Alliance
910 Seventeenth Street, NW, Suite 413
Washington, DC 20006
Phone: 202–331–1332
Fax: 202–331–2292
Web site: www.ovariancancer.org

SHARE
1501 Broadway, Suite 1720
New York, NY 10036
Phone: 212-719-0364 or 866-891-2392 toll free
Web site: www.sharecancersupport.org

Social Security Administration
Office of Public Inquiries
6401 Security Boulevard., Room 4-C–5 Annex
Baltimore, MD 21235–6401
Toll-free: 800–772–1213 or 800–325–0778 (TTY)
Web site: www.ssa.gov

Society of Gynecologic Oncologists
401 N. Michigan Avenue
Chicago, IL 60611
Phone: 312–644–6610
Web site: www.sgo.org

United Seniors Health Cooperative
409 Third Street SW, Suite 200
Washington, DC 20024
Phone: 202–479–6973
Toll-free: 800–637–2604
Web site: www.unitedseniorshealth.org

Online Resources

CancerNet (http://cancernet.nci.nih.gov)
  Detailed information on many types of cancer provided by the
  National Cancer Institute
Eyes on the Prize (www.eyesontheprize.org)
  A support community for women living with gynecologic
  cancer
Memorial Sloan-Kettering Cancer Center website
  (www.mskcc.org)
SHARE (www.sharecancersupport.org)
  A support community for women and their families living with
  breast or ovarian cancer.
Women's cancer network (www.wcn.org)
CancerLinks.org
CancerSource.com
CancerWise™ / MD Anderson Cancer Center web site:
  www.cancerwise.org
You Are Not Alone: www.yana.org
  Offers on-line and in-person support groups for those going
  through high-dose chemotherapy

Caregivers & Home Care

Family Caregiver Alliance
690 Market Street, Suite 600
San Francisco, CA 94104
Phone: 415-434-3388
Web site: www.caregiver.org
Caregiver resources include an online support group and an
information clearinghouse. Information available in Spanish.

National Family Caregivers Association
10400 Connecticut Avenue, #500
Kensington, MD 20895-3944
Phone: 800-896-3650
Web site: www.nfcacares.org
Provides education, information, support and advocacy services
for family caregivers.

CAREGIVERS (Association of Cancer Online Resources)
Web page: www.acor.org
Click on "Mailing Lists" and then select "CAREGIVERS."
Online discussion group for caregivers of cancer patients.

**Caring for the Caregiver (National Coalition for Cancer
Survivorship)**
Web page: www.cansearch.org/programs/Caregiver.PDF

**Guide for Cancer Supporters: Step-by-Step Ways to Help a
Relative or Friend Fight Cancer (R.A. Bloch Cancer
Foundation)**
Web page: www.blochcancer.org/guide/guidechp1.html

Children

Kids Konnected
27071 Cabot Road, Suite 102
Laguna Hills, CA 92653
Phone: 949-582-5443
Web site: *www.kidskonnected.org*
Provides extensive support resources and programs for children
who have a parent with cancer.

What Do I Tell the Children?—A Guide for a Parent with Cancer (CancerBACUP)
Web page: www.cancerbacup.org.uk/info/talk-children.htm

Clinical Trials Resources

There is no single resource for locating clinical trials for ovarian cancer. It makes sense to check all of the resources listed below repeatedly since new trials are continually added. There are also clinical trials services emerging that help to match patients to clinical trials. Some of these services can be useful for obtaining information and saving time, but it is important to read the company's privacy statement and be aware whether or not the company is being paid for recruiting patients before using them.

NCI Clinical Trials
Phone: 800-4CANCER
Web site: www.cancer.gov/clinical_trials/
The NCI offers comprehensive information on understanding and finding clinical trials, including access to the NCI/PDQ Clinical Trials Database.

NIH/NLM Clinical Trials
Web site: ClinicalTrials.gov
Clinical trials database service developed by the National Institute of Health's National Library of Medicine.

Centerwatch Clinical Trials Listing Service
Web site: www.centerwatch.com

Listing of Clinical Trials Conducted by Drug Companies.

NCI Clinical Trials and Insurance Coverage
Web page: cancertrials.nci.nih.gov/understanding/indepth/insurance/index.html
Excellent in-depth guide to clinical trials insurance issues.

Complementary & Alternative Medicine (CAM)

American Academy of Medical Acupuncture
Web site: www.medicalacupuncture.org
Professional site with articles on acupuncture, a list of frequently asked questions, and an acupuncturist locator.

Commonweal
P.O. Box 316
Bolinas, CA 94924
Phone: 415-868-0970
Web site: www.commonweal.org
Provides information on complementary approaches to cancer care, including the full-text of Michael Lerner's 1994 book, *Choices in Healing: Integrating the Best of Conventional and Complementary Approaches to Cancer,* published by MIT press (updated version available in print).

National Center for Complementary and Alternative Medicine (NCCAM)
Web site: nccam.nih.gov
Offers information on complementary and alternative medicine therapies, including NCI/PDQ expert-reviewed fact sheets on individual therapies and dietary supplements.

NCI Office of Cancer Complementary and Alternative Medicine (OCCAM)
Web site: www3.cancer.gov/occam
Information clearinghouse supporting the NCI's CAM activities.

Diet & Nutrition

American Institute for Cancer Research
1759 R Street, NW
Washington, DC 20009
Phone: 800-843-8114 | 202-328-7744 (in DC)
Web site: www.aicr.org
Supports research on diet and nutrition in the prevention and treatment of cancer. Provides information to cancer patients

on nutrition and cancer, including a compilation of healthy recipes. Maintains a nutrition hotline for questions relating to nutrition and health.

Nutrition (American Cancer Society)
Web page: www.cancer.org Enter "nutrition" in the search box.
Nutrition resources include: ACS guidelines on nutrition, dietary supplement information, nutrition message boards and tips on low-fat cooking and choosing healthy ingredients.

Drugs/Medications

MEDLINEplus: Drug Information
Web page: www.medlineplus.gov Click on the "drug information" button.
A guide to over 9,000 prescription and over-the-counter medications provided by U.S. Pharmacopeia (USP).

Employment, Insurance, Financial, & Legal Resources

Organizations and Programs

Americans with Disabilities Act (U.S. Department of Justice)
Web page: www.usdoj.gov/crt/ada/adahom1.htm
Cancer Legal Resource Center
919 S. Albany Street
Los Angeles, CA 90019-10015
Phone: 213-736-1455
A joint program of Loyola Law School and the Western Law Center for Disability Rights. Provides information and educational outreach on cancer-related legal issues to people with cancer and others impacted by the disease.

Centers for Medicare & Medicaid Services (CMS)
(formerly the Health Care Financing Administration [HCFA])
Web site: cms.hhs.gov
Oversees administration of:
• Medicare – federal health insurance program for people 65 years or older and some disabled people under 65 years.

Phone: 800-633-4227 | Web site: www.medicare.gov
- Medicaid – federal-state health insurance program for certain low-income people. Contact your state Medicaid offices for further information.

Web page: www.hcfa.gov/medicaid/medicaid.htm
- Health Insurance Portability and Accountability Act (HIPAA) - insurance reform that may lower your chance of losing existing coverage, ease your ability to switch health plans, and/or help you buy coverage on your own if you lose your employer's plan and have no other coverage available.

Web page: cms.hhs.gov. Enter "HIPAA" in the search box.

Family and Medical Leave Act (FMLA)

Web page: www.dol.gov/dol/esa/fmla.htm

U.S. Department of Labor web page providing information about the Family and Medical Leave Act (FMLA)

Health Insurance Association of America (HIAA)
1201 F Street, NW, Suite 500
Washington, DC 20004-1204
Phone: 202-824-1600
Web site: www.hiaa.org/cons/cons.htm
Provides insurance guides for consumers. Topics include health insurance and managed care, disability income, long-term care, and medical savings accounts.

Hill-Burton Program (Health Resources and Services Administration)

Phone: 301-443-5656 | 800-638-0742 (800-492-0359 in Maryland)
Web page: www.hrsa.gov:80/OSP/dfcr/obtain/obtain.htm
Facilities that receive Hill-Burton funds from the government are required by law to provide services to some people who cannot afford to pay. Information on Hill-Burton eligibility and facilities locations is available via phone or Internet.

Patient Advocate Foundation

753 Thimble Shoals Boulevard, Suite B
Newport News, VA 23606
Phone: 800-532-5274
Web site: www.patientadvocate.org

Nonprofit organization helps patients to resolve insurance, debt and job discrimination matters relative to cancer. Patient resources include: *The National Financial Resources Guidebook for Patient: A State-by-State Directory; Your Guide to the Appeals Process and the Managed Care Answer Guide,* among others.

Social Security Administration (SSA)

Web site: www.ssa.gov

Oversees two programs that pay benefits to people with disabilities:

- Social Security Disability Insurance - pays benefits to you and certain members of your family if you have worked long enough and paid Social Security taxes
- Supplemental Security Income – supplements Social Security payments based on need.

Veterans Health Administration

810 Vermont Avenue, NW
Washington, DC 20420
Phone: 202-273-5400 or 877-222-8387 (health care benefits)
Web site: www.va.gov/vbs/health/
Eligible veterans and their dependents may receive cancer treatment at a Veterans Administration Medical Center.

Financial Assistance Programs

Air Care Alliance

Phone: 888-260-9707
Web site: www.aircareall.org
Network of organizations willing to provide public benefit flights for health care.

Finding Ways to Pay for Care (National Coalition for Cancer Survivorship)

Web page: www.cansearch.org. Select "Programs" and then "Cancer Survival Toolbox".

NeedyMeds

Web site: www.needymeds.com
Information on patient assistance programs and other programs that help people obtain medications, supplies, and equipment.

Hospice & End-of-Life Issues

Partnership for Caring
1620 Eye Street, NW, Suite 202
Washington, DC 20006
Phone: 202-296-8071 | 800-989-9455
Web site: www.partnershipforcaring.org
Comprehensive information and resources covering end-of-life
    issues, including advanced directives.

CANCER-HOSPICE (Association of Online Cancer Resources)
Web site: www.acor.org. Click on "Mailing Lists" and then select
    "CANCER-HOSPICE."
Online discussion group for cancer patients dealing with hospice
    issues.

Growth House
Web site: www.growthhouse.org
Extensive, annotated directory to hospice and end-of-life
    resources. Organized by topic.

Home Care Guide for Advanced Cancer (American College of Physicians)
Web page: www.acponline.org/public/h_care/
Guide for family and friends caring for advanced cancer patients
    who are living at home.

Hospice Net
Web site: www.hospicenet.org
Provides comprehensive information to patients and families fac-
    ing life-threatening illness. Extensive resources addressing end-
    of-life issues from both patient and caregiver perspectives.

Patient Advocacy Skills
Cancer Survival Toolbox (National Coalition for Cancer
    Survivorship)
Web page: www.cansearch.org. Select "Programs" and then
    "Cancer Survival Toolbox."
Topics include: communication skills, finding information, solv-
    ing problems, making decisions, negotiating and standing up
    for your rights. (Also available as audiotapes at 877-866-
    5748.)

Physician & Hospital Locators

American Society of Clinical Oncology (ASCO)
Web page: www.asco.org. Click on the "Find an Oncologist"
button.

American College of Surgeons (ACS) Commission on Cancer
Web page: www.facs.org/public_info/yourhealth/aahcp.html
Listing of ACS Commission on Cancer's Approved Hospital
Cancer Programs.

American Medical Association (AMA) Physician Select
Web page: www.ama-assn.org/aps/amahg.htm
Provides professional information on licensed U.S. physicians.

Prevention & Risk Assessment

Prevention (American Cancer Society)
Web page: www.cancer.org. Enter "prevention" in the search box.
Comprehensive section on prevention covers topics such as environmental and occupational cancer risks, exercise, tobacco and
cancer, nutrition for risk reduction, and prevention and detection programs.

Your Cancer Risk (Harvard Center for Cancer Prevention)
Web site: www.yourcancerrisk.harvard.edu
Online ovarian cancer risk assessment tool.

Research Resources & Reference

PubMed: MEDLINE (National Library of Medicine)
Web site: www.ncbi.nlm.nih.gov/PubMed/
Provides free online access to MEDLINE, a database of over
11 million citations to the medical literature.

Medscape
Web site: www.medscape.com. Enter "ovarian cancer" in the
search box.
Medscape is an excellent source for the latest news in lung cancer
research, including access to summaries of cancer conferences.
Aimed at health care professionals. Registration required for
free access to Medscape.

Appendix

Merriam Webster Medical Dictionary
Web site: www.intelihealth.com. Enter "Merriam Webster" in
the search box.
Registration required for free access to Intelihealth.

Support Services

Association of Cancer Online Resources (ACOR)
Web site: www.acor.org. Click on "Mailing Lists."
ACOR offers online support groups for cancer patients.

Cancer Care
275 Seventh Avenue
New York, NY 10001
Phone: 212-712-8080 | 800-813-4673
Web site: www.cancercare.org
Provides comprehensive support services and programs to people
with cancer.

Cancer Survivors Network
Web site: www.acscsn.org
ACSCSN is the American Cancer Society's online patient
community.

R.A. Bloch National Cancer Foundation
4400 Main Street
Kansas City, MO 64111
Phone: 816-932-8453 or 800-433-0464
Web site: www.blochcancer.org
Provides Bloch-authored cancer books free of charge, a multidis-
ciplinary referral service and patient-to-patient phone support.

Vital Options International
15060 Ventura Boulevard, Suite 211
Sherman Oaks, CA 91403
Phone: 818-788-5225
Web site: www.vitaloptions.org
Produces "The Group Room," a weekly, syndicated radio call-in
show (with simultaneous webcast) covering important and
timely topics in cancer.

Wellness Community
35 East Seventh Street, Suite 412
Cincinnati, OH 45202
Phone: 513-421-7111 or 888-793-WELL
Web site: www.wellness-community.org
Provides educational programs and support groups for people
    with cancer and their families.

Talking About Cancer (American Cancer Society)
Web page: www.cancer.org. Enter "Talking About Cancer" in
    the search box.
Discusses how to talk about your cancer with family, friends, your
    health care providers and your employer. Includes resources for
    locating in-person and online support groups.
Coping with Cancer. Cancer magazine available free of charge in
    oncology offices or by subscription at 615-791-3859 or
    www.copingmag.com

Symptoms, Side Effects, & Complications

Fatigue
CancerFatigue.org
Web site: www.cancerfatigue.org
Information about cancer-related fatigue for patients and
    caregivers.

**CANCER-FATIGUE (Association of Cancer Online
Resources)**
Web page: www.acor.org. Click on "Mailing Lists" and then
    select "CANCER-FATIGUE."
Online discussion list covering cancer and treatment-related
    fatigue.

**NCCN Cancer-Related Fatigue Treatment Guidelines for
Patients**
Web page:
    www.nccn.org/patient_gls/_english/_fatigue/index.htm

Appendix

Nausea and Vomiting

NCCN Nausea and Vomiting Treatment Guidelines for Patients with Cancer
Web page:
www.nccn.org/patient_gls/_english/_nausea_and_vomiting/index.htm

NCI/PDQ Nausea and Vomiting
Web page: cancer.gov Enter "nausea" in the search box.
Expert-reviewed information summary about cancer-related nausea and vomiting.

Nutritional Problems

NCI/PDQ Nutrition
Web site: cancer.gov. Enter "nutrition" in the search box.
Expert-reviewed information summary about the causes and management of nutritional problems occurring in cancer patients.

Pain

The National Pain Foundation (NPF)
P.O. Box 102605
Denver, CO 80250-2605
Web site: www.painconnection.org
NFP web site offers online education and support communities for pain patients and their families, including cancer pain and palliative care resources.

CANCER-PAIN (Association of Cancer Online Resources)
Web page: www.acor.org. Click on "Mailing Lists" and then select "CANCER-PAIN."
Online discussion list about pain associated with cancer and its treatments.

NCCN Cancer Pain Treatment Guidelines for Patients
Web page: www.nccn.org/patient_gls/_english/_pain/index.htm

NCI/PDQ Pain

Web page: cancer.gov. Enter "pain" in the search box.

Expert-reviewed information summary about cancer-related pain. Includes discussion of approaches to the management and treatment of cancer-associated pain.

Peripheral Neuropathy

The Neuropathy Association

60 East 42nd Street, Suite 942

New York, NY 10165

Phone: 212-692-0662

Web site: www.neuropathy.org

CANCER-NEUROPATHY (Association of Cancer Online Resources)

Web page: www.acor.org   Click on "Mailing Lists" and then select "CANCER-NEUROPATHY."

Online discussion group for patients dealing with neuropathy induced by cancer or its treatments.

Almadrones, L.A. and R. Arcot. "Patient Guide to Peripheral Neuropathy." Oncology Nursing Forum 26, no. 8 (1999): 1359-1362.

Pleural Effusion

Chemical Pleurodesis for Malignant Pleural Effusion (Cancer Supportive Care)

Web page: www.cancersupportivecare.com/pleural.html

Carolyn Clary-Macy, RN, provides a clear explanation of chemical pleurodesis for malignant pleural effusion. Aimed at patients.

Sexual Effects

CANCER-FERTILITY & CANCER-SEXUALITY (Association of Cancer Online Resources)

Web site: www.acor.org. Click on "Mailing Lists." and then select "CANCER-FERTILITY" and/or "CANCER-SEXUALITY."

Online discussion lists about fertility and sexuality issues associated with cancer.

Appendix

NCI/PDQ Sexuality and Reproductive Issues
Web page: cancer.gov. Enter "sexuality" in the search box.
Expert-reviewed information summary about factors that may
affect fertility and sexual functioning in people who have
cancer.

Tests & Procedures

Diagnostic Imaging (MEDLINEplus)
Web page:
www.nlm.nih.gov/medlineplus/diagnosticimaging.html

Laboratory Tests (MEDLINEplus)
Web page: www.nlm.nih.gov/medlineplus/laboratorytests.html
Margolis, Simeon, ed. 2001. *The Johns Hopkins Consumer Guide to
Medical Tests: What You Can Expect, How You Should Prepare,
What Your Results Mean.* Baltimore, MD: The Johns Hopkins
University Press.

Treatment Information & Guidelines

Chemotherapy and You (NIH/NCI)
Web page: cancer.gov. Enter "Chemotherapy and You" in the
search box. Also available in print by calling 800-4CANCER.

Radiation Therapy and You (NIH/NCI)
Web page: cancer.gov. Enter "Radiation Therapy and You"
in the search box. Also available in print by calling
800-4CANCER.

Survivorship Issues

LT-SURVIVORS (Association of Cancer Online Resources)
Web page: www.acor.org. Click on "Mailing Lists" and then
select "LT-SURVIVORS."
Forum for discussion of issues of concern to long-term cancer
survivors.

Books and Pamphlets

The following books are available from the American Cancer Society:

The American Cancer Society's Guide to Pain Control: Powerful Methods to Overcome Cancer Pain
Coming to Terms with Cancer
Informed Decisions, 2nd Edition
American Cancer Society's Guide to Complementary and Alternative Cancer Methods
Caregiving
Women and Cancer

The following pamphlets are available from the National Cancer Institute:

Chemotherapy and You: A Guide to Self-Help During Treatment
Eating Hints for Cancer Patients Before, During, and After Treatment
Get Relief from Cancer Pain
Helping Yourself During Chemotherapy
Questions and Answers About Pain Control: A Guide for People with Cancer and Their Families
Taking Time: Support for People with Cancer and the People Who Care About Them
Taking Part in Clinical Trials: What Cancer Patients Need to Know

Available in Spanish:

Datos sobre el tratamiento de quimioterapia contra el cancer
El tratamiento de radioterapia; guia para el paciente durante el tratamiento
En que consisten los estudios clinicos? Un folleto para los pacientes de cancer

The following pamphlets are available from the National Comprehensive Cancer Network:

Cancer Pain Treatment Guidelines for Patients
Nausea and Vomiting Treatment Guidelines for Patient with Cancer

Appendix

Available in Spanish:
El dolor asociado con el cáncer

Available from The Wellness Community:
A Patient Active Guide to Living With Ovarian Cancer.

Abrahm JL. A Physician's Guide to Pain and Symptom Management in Cancer Patients. Baltimore: Johns Hopkins University Press, 2000.

American Cancer Society's Guide to Complementary and Alternative Cancer Methods. Atlanta, GA: American Cancer Society, 2000.

Anderson, G. 50 Essential Things to Do When the Doctor Says It's Cancer. New York: Penguin Books, 1993.

Benson, H. The Relaxation Response. New York: Avon Books, 1975.

Carney KL. What is Cancer Anyway? Explaining Cancer to Children of All Ages. Dragonfly Publishing, 1998.

Cassileth, BR. The Alternative Medicine Handbook: The Complete Reference Guide to Alternative and Complementary Therapies. New York: W.W. Norton & Company, 1998.

Conner K, Langford L, Mayer M. Ovarian Cancer: Your Guide to Taking Control. Patient-Centered Guides, 2003.

Consumers Guide to Cancer Drugs. Atlanta, GA: American Cancer Society, 2000.

Finn, R. Cancer Clinical Trials: Experimental Treatments & How They Can Help You. Sebastopol, CA: O'Reilly & Associates, 1999.

Hapham WH. When a Parent Has Cancer: A Guide to Caring for Your Children. HarperCollins, 1997.

Harpham, WS. "Resolving the Frustration of Fatigue." CA: A Cancer Journal for Clinicians. 1999; 49: 178-189.

Harpham, WS. After Cancer: A Guide to Your New Life. New York: W.W. Norton & Company, 1994.

Hoffman, B. Working It Out: Your Employment Rights as a Cancer Survivor. Silver Spring, MD: National Coalition for Cancer Survivorship, undated. This booklet can be ordered from the NCCS at 877-622-7937.

Holland, JC. and Sheldon Lewis. The Human Side of Cancer. New York: HarperCollins Publishers, 2000.

Houts, PS. and Bucher, JA, eds. Caregiving: A Step-by-Step Resource for Caring for the Person with Cancer at Home. Atlanta, GA: American Cancer Society, 2000.

Kalter S. 1987. Looking Up: The Complete Guide to Looking and Feeling Good for the Recovering Cancer Patient. Provides tips (with photos) on hair care, wigs, makeup, and exercise. (Out of print; check your local library to find a copy.)

Kaptchuk, TJ. The Web That Has No Weaver: Understanding Chinese Medicine. McGraw-Hill, 2000.

Kohlenberg S. 1993. Sammy's Mommy Has Cancer.

Landay, DS. Be Prepared: The Complete Financial, Legal and Practical Guide to Living with Cancer, HIV and Other Life-Challenging Conditions. New York: St. Martin's Press, 1998.

Laughlin, EH. Coming to Terms with Cancer: A Glossary of Cancer-Related Terms Atlanta, GA: American Cancer Society, 2002.

McKay, J and Hirano, N. The Chemotherapy and Radiation Therapy Survival Guide. Oakland, CA: New Harbinger Publications, Inc., 1998.

Mulay M. 2002. Making the Decision: A Cancer Patient's Guide to Clinical Trials. Sudbury, MA: Jones & Bartlett Publishers, 2002.

Olson, K. Surgery and Recovery. Traverse City, MI: Rhodes & Easton, 1998.

Oster, N et al. Making Informed Medical Decisions: Where to Look and How to Use What You Find. Sebastapol, CA: O'Reilly & Associates, Inc., 2000.

Outstanding article by a patient/physician discusses cancer-related fatigue and how to deal with it.

Piver MS, Wilder G, Bull J. 1998. Gilda's Disease: Sharing Personal Experiences and a Medical Perspective on Ovarian Cancer. Bantam Doubleday, 1998.

Schimmel, S.R., and Fox, B. Cancer Talk: Voices of Hope and Endurance from "The Group Room," the World's Largest Cancer Support Group. New York: Broadway Books, 1999.

Willis, Joanie. The Cancer Patient's Workbook. New York: Dorling Kindersley Publishing, Inc., 2001.

Appendix

Glossary

Adenocarcinomas: Type of cancer, arising from the cells of epithelial origin.

Adenomas: Noncancerous tumors arising from epithelial cells.

Adhesions: Scarring within the abdominal cavity that commonly occurs after surgery.

Adjuvant: Given after a primary procedure.

Anechoic: Used in ultrasound studies, describes a lack of different ultrasound signals, commonly seen with simple cysts.

Antiangiogenesis: To block new blood vessel formation.

Antigen: A protein that sits on or is released from cells that can be targeted with an antibody or vaccine.

Antihistamine: To block the release of histamines, which are often associated with allergic reactions.

Apoptosis: Programmed cell death.

Ascites: Fluid build-up within the abdomen.

Atypia: Used by pathologists, it describes abnormal cellular changes seen under the microscope.

Belly wash: Common term for an intraperitoneal treatment.

Benign: Not cancerous.

Bilateral salpingo-oophorectomy: The surgical term for removal of both the right and left fallopian tubes and ovaries.

Biopsy: Small amount of tissue taken during surgery or a less invasive procedure for analysis by a pathologist.

Borderline: A term used to describe a tumor that does not appear normal but does not meet a pathologist's criteria for cancer; otherwise described as low malignant potential.

Bowel obstruction: Condition where the small or large bowel is blocked, due to either adhesions or tumor that causes the bowel to back up instead of work normally (to get rid of stool).

Capillaries: The smallest blood vessels within your body.

Carbohydrate antigen: A type of protein released from cells.

Carcinomatosis: Cancer deposits along the abdomen, often along the bowel and involving the omentum.

Clinical complete remission: A normal physical exam, tumor marker, and radiology tests following the completion of treatment for cancer.

Cognitive: Referring to brain function.

Colon: The large intestine, part of your gastrointestinal tract. The function is to absorb water and food and to excrete stool.

Colonic dilation: The end process of a bowel obstruction where in the bowel essentially bursts because neither food or gas can move.

Colostomy: Loop of bowel that is pulled through your skin.

Complete resection: Removal of all the tumor in your abdomen and pelvis.

Computed tomography: Otherwise known as a CT scan, this is a highly sensitive radiology exam used to help diagnose and follow patients with cancer.

Cremaphore: A molecule to which drugs are attached to increase the drug's delivery into your body.

Cytological analysis: The process of examining cells under the microscope, which are usually obtained from floating cells in the fluid of the abdomen (ascites) or chest (pleural effusions).

Debulking: The process of removing cancer from your body.

Differentiation: The process of cells maturing so they can perform specific processes in our bodies.

Direct extension: The process by which cancer extends into local and surrounding tissue.

Dyspnea: Shortness of breath.

Early satiety: Feeling of getting full faster than you normally would.

Echogenic: An ultrasound term describing complex patterns seen within a cyst.

Endodermal sinus tumor: A type of germ cell tumor, derived from early cells destined to become eggs. Otherwise, they are referred to as **yolk-sac tumors**.

Endoscopic camera: A flexible camera within a tube (the endoscope) that is used to do minimally invasive procedures.

Estrogen: A female hormone produced by the ovaries; it is responsible for female changes during maturity.

First-degree relatives: Blood relatives of your immediate family (father, mother, sister, or brother).

Fistulas: Abnormally formed channels between two otherwise separate organs, such as between the vagina and bladder (vesicovaginal) or between the bowel and the skin (enterocutaneous).

Gastroenterologist: A medical specialist in treating disorders of the esophagus, stomach, bowel, and rectum.

Genomics: The study of gene expression patterns.

Grade: A pathologist term that defines how abnormal a cell is under the microscope.

Gynecological oncologist: A specialist in the treatment of cancer of the female reproductive system.

Hematogenous dissemination: A process of spread by which cancer travels through the bloodstream.

Hydronephrosis: Abnormal enlargement of the kidney.

Hydroureteronephrosis: Abnormal enlargement of the kidney and the tube where urine flows, called the ureter.

Intraperitoneal: Into the abdomen.

Intraperitoneal port: A surgically placed device placed under the skin and into the abdomen that allows directed treatment into the abdomen.

Intubation: Process by which a person is placed on a breathing machine.

Krukenberg tumor: A cancer that has gone into the ovary from another place, usually starting in the stomach.

Laparoscopy: Camera-directed surgery done without creating a large incision into the abdomen.

Laparotomy: Surgery through a large incision into the abdomen.

Letrozole: An anti-estrogen medication.

Leuprolide acetate: An anti-hormone which blocks release of estrogen and progesterone at the level of the brain.

Lymphatic channels: Vessels through which lymph fluid travels; part of the lymphatic system.

Lymphatic spread: Metastasis of cancer cells through the lymphatic system.

Lymphatic system: A network of lymphatic channels, lymph nodes, and organs such as the spleen and the tonsils that are the major component of the immune system.

Menopause: Physical changes marking the end of a woman's fertile years, the most notable being the cessation of the menstrual cycles.

Menstruation: Vaginal bleeding due to endometrial shedding following ovulation when the egg is not fertilized.

Metastases: Tumor that has spread to distant places in the body.

Metastatic: Adjective used to describe tumor that has spread.

Mitosis: Process of cells dividing.

Mixed mesodermal tumors: Tumors of dual origin with one part consisting of carcinomas and the other part consisting of sarcoma, hence their other designation as a carcinosarcoma.

Moderately differentiated: A pathologist's term to describe cellular changes of a cancer cell; this describes cells that do not resemble the normal appearance but are still recognizable as related to their normal counterpart.

Multicompartmental: Multiple spaces, used to describe a finding seen in complex cysts seen on imaging studies, like ultrasounds.

Mutations: Genetic changes in DNA; mutations are not always harmful but sometimes can be associated with cancer development.

Nasogastric (NG) tube: A tube placed temporarily through the nose (naso) into the stomach (gastric) to help relieve continuous vomiting caused by a bowel obstruction.

Neoadjuvant treatment: Treatment given before surgery.

Omental cake: Tumor involvement of the omentum that results in the formation of a large mass.

Omentum: Lining of the small and large bowels.

Ovulation: Process of egg release from the ovary.

Palliation: To provide relief of pain. Adj: Palliative.

Papilla: Budding formations on structures, seen on ultrasound or other imaging.

Paracentesis: The process of removing ascites.

Pathological remission: The finding of no residual cancer at the end of primary treatment for cancer; only diagnosed in a second surgical procedure.

Patient-controlled analgesia (PCA): A method of providing pain medication through the vein that allows direct control over the amount required to make one comfortable.

Percutaneous endoscopic gastrostomy (PEG): A tube placed by a gastroenterologist that is inserted through your skin (percutaneous) and into your stomach using a flexible tube containing a camera (endoscopic). A hole is made in the stomach (gastrotomy) and the tube is fixed from the stomach and exits the skin. The purpose is to allow continuous drainage of bowel contents in a woman with terminal cancer who has an intractable bowel obstruction.

Perforation: Bowel injury where a hole is caused, usually as a result of bowel obstruction, surgery, or infection.

Performance status: A numerical description of how a person is doing in their normal day-to-day life and whether their cancer is impacting on their ability to live normally.

Peritoneal carcinomatosis: Involvement of the omentum or bowels with cancer, usually at the size of "rice granules" or tumor nodules.

Peritoneal cavity: The abdominal space.

Peritoneal seeding: Process of cancer spreading to involve the peritoneal surface.

Peritoneovenous shunt: Device that allows drainage of ascites from the peritoneum directly back into the bloodstream.

Peritoneum: The lining of the peritoneal cavity.

Pleural effusion: Fluid build-up around the lungs.

Pleurodesis: Process performed to prevent further build-up of fluid around the lung.

Poorly differentiated: A pathologist's term to describe cellular changes of a cancer cell; this describes cells that bear no resemblance to their normal counterpart.

Primary peritoneal cancer: Cancer that arises from the lining of the gut, or the peritoneum. This cancer behaves similarly to ovarian cancer, and is treated much in the same way.

Prognosis: An estimate of the outlook following the diagnosis of a disease such as cancer.

Prophylactic oophorectomy: Removal of a woman's eggs in an attempt to reduce or remove a risk for cancer in the future.

Proteomics: The study of protein profiles.

Pulmonary fibrosis: Scarring of the lung tissue, which is generally not reversible.

Regeneration: To grow back.

Renin: A hormone released by the kidney normally which is important in maintaining hydration.

Reservoir: A receptacle that holds fluid.

Second-line chemotherapy: Chemotherapy given during recurrence.

Sensory neuropathy: Numbness and tingling, usually involving the hands and feet.

Septations: Thin membranes or walls dividing an area into multiple chambers. Often used to describe complex cysts seen on ultrasound.

Serological relapse: Diagnosis of recurrence solely based on an elevation of a tumor marker without evidence of recurrence by radiology tests.

Sporadic: Isolated; to occur without a pattern.

Suboptimal debulking: Residual disease greater than 1 cm in diameter upon completion of surgery.

Surgical staging: Procedure of determining the extent of cancer present.

T-cells: Cells involved in our immune system.

Theca-lutein cysts: Functional cysts that occur in the ovary due to the cyclic changes of hormones during a woman's period.

Thoracentesis: Procedure of draining a pleural effusion.

Thoracic surgeon: A surgeon who has completed extra training in the surgical management of diseases involving the chest and its organs.

Torsion: Act of twisting or turning in on itself (ovarian torsion, for example).

Total hysterectomy: Surgical excision of the uterus and cervix.

Total parenteral nutrition (TPN): Nutrition that is given by vein.

Treatment-free interval: The time between the end of one chemotherapy regimen to initiation of a subsequent therapy for recurrent disease.

Treatment holiday: A break in treatment that allows the body time to recover from toxicity.

True negative rate: The proportion of patients who have a negative test result and who do not have the disease.

True positive rate: The proportion of patients who have positive test results and who do have the disease.

Tumor: A mass of cells that grow abnormally.

Undifferentiated: A pathologist term to describe cellular changes of a cancer cell; this describes cells that bear no resemblance at all to normal cells.

Ureters: The anatomical structure that enables us to get rid of urine. It connects the kidney to the bladder.

Vaccine: A preparation that is given to induce immunity to a disease or condition.

Well-differentiated: A pathologist's term to describe cellular changes of a cancer cell; this describes cells that meet criteria for cancer but still maintain a resemblance to normal cells.

Index